Edgar Cayce's I

Optimal
and Weight Loss

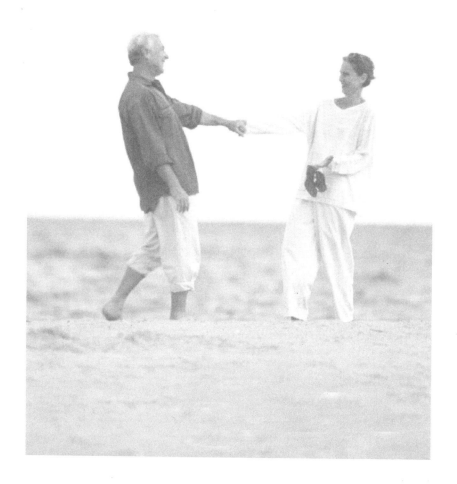

Edgar Cayce's Diet Plan for

Optimal Health
and Weight Loss

By
Simone Gabbay

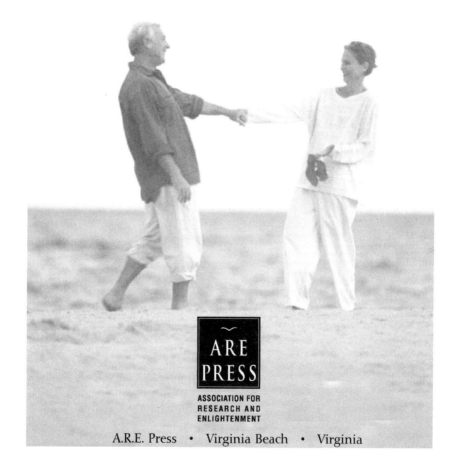

~
ARE
PRESS

ASSOCIATION FOR
RESEARCH AND
ENLIGHTENMENT

A.R.E. Press • Virginia Beach • Virginia

A.R.E. Press
215 67th Street
Virginia Beach, VA 23451-2061

Library of Congress Cataloging-in-Publication Data
Gabbay, Simone, 1956–
    Edgar Cayce's diet plan for optimal health and weight loss / by
Simone Gabbay.
        p. cm.
    Includes index.
    ISBN 13: 978-0-87604-564-0 (trade paper)
    1. Cayce, Edgar, 1877-1945. 2. Nutrition. 3. Weight loss. I. Title.
    RA784.G297 2007
                                                2007042673

A Note to the Reader:
No part of this book is intended to substitute for competent medical diagnosis, nor does the A.R.E. endorse any of the information contained herein as prescription for the treatment of disease. Edgar Cayce gave health readings for particular individuals with specific conditions; therefore, any application of his advice in present–day treatment planning should be undertaken only after consulting with a professional practitioner in a related field. It is especially important that you do not discontinue any prescribed treatment without the full concurrence of your doctor.

Cover design by Richard Boyle

Table of Contents

Introduction
Edgar Cayce's Legacy of Health and Healing ix

Chapter 1
A Weighty Challenge 1
 • Malnourished heavyweights 4
 • Battle the bulge while you can 5
 • Choosing a diet that fits 6
 • South Beach and Cayce 7

Chapter 2
Give Me Five: The Principles of Healthy Eating 10
 • Cayce diet 101: keeping the body alkaline 11
 • Five principles of healthy eating 14

Chapter 3
Indulge in Water 17
Healthy Eating Principle No. 1
 • Water + walking = weight loss 19
 • Choosing your drinking water 19
 • Shun sugary soft drinks 21

Chapter 4
Favor Veggies and Fruits 23
Healthy Eating Principle No. 2
 • Enzymes in raw vegetables and fruits 26
 • Fresh juice power 29
 • Ready for a juice fast? 31
 • Crunchy crucifers 32
 • Jerusalem artichokes 34
 • Nutritious sea veggies 36
 • The art of gentle cookery 39
 • Fruits for your health 41
 • Grapes and grape juice—nature's
   prescription for weight loss 43

• Keeping your veggies and fruits fresh 46
• Preserving vegetables and fruits:
  canning, freezing, drying, and fermenting 48
• Locally grown and seasonal foods 51
• Above and below ground 52
• Why eat organic? 53

Chapter 5
Prioritize for Protein 58
Healthy Eating Principle No. 3
• A fresh look at whole eggs 59
• Milk in the making 61
• Fowl–the meat of choice 64
• Dangers of processed meats 66
• Fish failings 66
• Be soy sensible 68

Chapter 6
Keep Starches in Check 70
Healthy Eating Principle No. 4
• What's in a grain kernel? 71
• The glycemic index 72
• Alternative grains 74
• Think whole salt 75
• Naturally sweet and wholesome 76
• Breakfast: an epiphany 78

Chapter 7
Banish Fake Fats 80
Healthy Eating Principle No. 5
• Butter is better 82
• Olive oil–queen among oils 83
• Beware of fake oils 85
• Fats that boost metabolism 85
• Healthy and nutty 86

Chapter 8
Treats to Slim Down With 88
  • Fruit and veggie power 88
  • Nuts, seeds, and cereal bars 89
  • Edgar Cayce's Mummy Food 89
  • Easy snacks 91
  • Chocolate: a new health food? 91

Chapter 9
Get Physical–The Surefire Way to Burn Fat Fast 93
  • Walk weight away 95
  • Optimize your workout–take a deep breath 98
  • Warm up to stretching 100
  • Eating for a great workout 102
  • Clearing cellulite naturally 104

Chapter 10
Taming Stress 111
  • Stress-free eating 113
  • Get your sleep to lose your weight 114
  • Planning better sleep 116

Chapter Summary
Getting Started on Your Cayce Diet and Health Program 119
  • Should you take supplements? 124
  • Affirmation for weight loss 127

Recipes Section 128

Internet Resources 151

Index 153

Introduction

Edgar Cayce's Legacy of Health and Healing

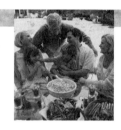

THE NATURAL HEALTH AND WEIGHT-LOSS RECOMMENDATIONS outlined in this book are based on the work of the late Edgar Cayce, one of the greatest visionaries of all time. For more than a hundred years, Cayce's work has been the focus of interest and research for individuals, groups, and professionals from around the world. His psychic readings, painstakingly documented and clinically tested by many dedicated individuals and groups, have helped thousands achieve better health and well-being. Moreover, as will become evident throughout this book, there is today increasing validation of the readings by a growing body of mainstream scientific research.

Edgar Cayce's unusual gift was discovered in his early twenties, when a hypnotherapist whom he had consulted for a condition marked by the loss of his voice was amazed that Cayce, in a hypnotic state, accurately diagnosed the cause of his own problem. The condition, medically classified as *aphonia*, had not responded to treatment by any doctor. During the session with the hypnotherapist, the young Cayce spoke in a normal voice, explaining that the illness was psychosomatic and had been caused by nervous tension. He went on to recommend that he be given the hypnotic suggestion to increase circulation to the affected area, which would serve to normalize the condition. To everyone's surprise, this "treatment" was effective, and Cayce fully regained the use of his voice.

The hypnotherapist, who was also a student of osteopathy and a self-taught practitioner of suggestive therapeutics, was so impressed with the remarkable results of the experiment that he decided to try out the young Cayce's newly discovered diagnostic powers on some of his clients who had failed to receive help from conventional medical doctors. Time and again, the results proved impressive, demonstrating accuracy in diagnosis and surprising success in the application of the recommended treatment protocols.

The role of psychic diagnostician was an unusual vocation for Edgar Cayce that he had not consciously chosen or planned. Deeply committed to his Christian faith, the young Edgar, who was born in 1877 near Hopkinsville, Kentucky, had aspired to entering the ministry, but was unable to pursue formal theological studies due to lack of money. He became a devoted Sunday School teacher instead. His love of the Bible was demonstrated in the fact that he read it from cover to cover once for every year of his life.

In his childhood, he displayed special gifts, for instance, when he was able, on occasion, to communicate with those who had passed on. His favorite playmates were other-dimensional beings, such as elves or fairies. At the age of thirteen, Edgar Cayce had a most remarkable experience that appears to have set the stage for his life's work: A beautiful woman appeared to him in a vision and asked him what he most wished for in his life. He answered that more than anything, he wanted to help others, especially children who were ill. Shortly thereafter, the young Edgar developed a highly unusual talent: he was able to sleep on a book and, on awakening, remember its entire contents. While this remarkable ability helped him improve his school grades for some time, it eventually faded. However, it appears that the true fulfillment of his wish to help others became manifest in his work as a psychic and visionary, on a scale that was many times larger than he could ever have imagined.

In his self-induced hypnotic state, Cayce had the uncanny ability to allow his mind to travel anywhere in space and time. He was able to telepathically scan another person's body and accurately determine its condition, along with symptoms and their causes, and to recommend therapies and remedies that would help correct any ailments that were identified. This ability was all the more remarkable because, in his trance state, Cayce made use of medical terminology that he could not even understand while awake. Equally amazing was the fact that the whereabouts of the person being examined were irrelevant—he or she could be in the same room with Cayce or going about activities in another town or country—the information being sought for that person was equally accessible to Cayce.

Nearly two-thirds of the readings Cayce gave in his lifetime addressed health and medical concerns. The therapeutic recommendations made by the sleeping Cayce were consistently holistic, meaning that they touched on the mental, emotional, and spiritual aspects of a person as much as the physical. One of the essential concepts from the readings is that *spirit is life; the mind is the builder; the physical is the result.* It was through the lens of this paradigm that the suggestions in the readings were offered.

For several years, Cayce refused to accept compensation for his readings, not wanting to use for personal gain a gift he had received from God. He provided a modest living for himself and his family through his work as a professional photographer. Eventually, however, the growing number of requests for readings forced him to dedicate himself to this calling on a full-time basis. Cayce went on to give more than fourteen thousand psychic readings on hundreds of subjects ranging from diverse health concerns to the origins of the universe and the spiritual evolution of the human race. These readings were stenographically recorded by his devoted secretary, Gladys Davis. Now fully cataloged, they are available in searchable electronic format (EdgarCayce.org) through the Association for Research and Enlightenment (A.R.E.) in Virginia Beach, Virginia, where Cayce and his family settled in 1925.

In the ensuing years, as Cayce's fame grew nationwide and demand for the readings soared, there were medical professionals among his supporters who worked with the suggestions from the readings. One of the most influential for the future of Cayce's work was Dr. Harold J. Reilly, a physiotherapist, chiropractor, and naturopath. Although he and Edgar Cayce had never heard of each other, Reilly was singled out in the readings as the health professional best able to carry out many of the prescribed treatments. In 1930, when patients started coming to his practice in New York with referrals from Edgar Cayce, Reilly was surprised to find that the diagnoses and treatment recommendations the patients brought with them originated in psychic readings. The material presented by the patients seemed plausible enough, however, for the open-minded Reilly to carry out Cayce's instructions. Encouraged by the positive results of the treatments, Reilly became fascinated with the phenomenon of the psychic diagnostician and began a lifelong study of the readings. After the closure of his famous Reilly Health Institute in Rockefeller Center in 1965, Harold Reilly set up a physiotherapy clinic in Virginia Beach—the forerunner of today's A.R.E. Health Center and Spa.

Dr. Reilly passed away in 1987 at the age of 92, but his classic bestseller, *The Edgar Cayce Handbook for Health Through Drugless Therapy*, continues to educate its readers in the practical knowledge of Cayce's health programs, medically tested by the health professional who was specially chosen in the readings. Reilly's name and work also live on in the Cayce/Reilly® School of Massotherapy, whose facilities are located in the original hospital building of the A.R.E. in Virginia Beach. The school provides professional training for massage therapists and offers a variety of holistic studies.

Dr. William A. McGarey is another medical pioneer who has worked extensively with the health information from the Cayce readings. An internationally acclaimed physician and the author of several books based on the Cayce material, McGarey is also co-founder of the A.R.E. Clinic in Phoenix, Arizona, which continues to make Cayce therapies and treatment protocols available to the public. Now in his late 80s, Dr. Bill, as he is affectionately known to his many friends, has retired from active medical practice. However, his writings and teachings continue to inspire Cayce fans worldwide.

In the twenty-first century, the health information from the Cayce readings remains an enormous resource for medical professionals interested in applying holistic medicine at its best and for all individuals looking to achieve optimal health and well-being for themselves and their loved ones.

One of the most widely discussed and applied areas of research from the readings is the large body of information on diet and nutrition. For nearly every ailment Cayce was asked about, he suggested dietary adjustments. Although much of the readings' nutritional advice was given for individuals with differing biochemical constitutions and specific pathological conditions, there are many common elements that form the basis of what students of the readings have termed *the Cayce diet*.

The Cayce diet is not specifically a weight-loss diet, although many who have adopted it have found that gradual, long-term weight loss is one of its surprising side effects. Rather, the diet represents a way of eating that optimizes nutrient intake and assimilation and enhances all metabolic functions and processes, including the body's ability to burn fat.

This was the experience of Catherine MacDonald of Bracebridge, Ontario, Canada: "When my husband and I switched over to the alkaline-forming Cayce diet for his arthritis," says Catherine, "I lost about twenty pounds and have been able to keep it off by staying on the diet." Her husband, James Schmidt, who also lost several pounds after adopting the Cayce protocol for arthritis (with outstanding success), says that the alkaline diet has been instrumental in helping him maintain a healthy, stable weight over the past seven years.

Nancy Thomas of Elmwood, Ontario, Canada, has also found the Cayce diet tremendously helpful in her recovery from chronic illness, as well as in balancing her weight: "The Cayce alkaline/acid balance diet was imperative for my recovery from chronic fatigue and fibromyalgia," she says. "The use of castor oil packs and following a low-acid diet seem to be the answer to losing weight, health maintenance, and the prevention of colds and flu. It works!"

When digestion and nutrient assimilation improve and all metabolic processes are restored to optimal function, the natural result is a healthier, leaner body, abundant in energy and well-being.

The dietary guidelines from the Edgar Cayce readings do not require us to count calories nor measure grams of fat nor calculate a body mass index. They simply provide us with an understanding of healthful eating—a diet plan based on natural whole foods set in the context of a spiritual universe.

I pray and trust that the information contained in this book will also help you find good health, happiness, and your ideal body weight.

1

A Weighty Challenge

IF WE BELIEVED THE HEADLINES on the covers of some popular magazines, then weight loss would simply be a matter of consuming a miracle food or supplement that could magically melt off several pounds in a mere week or weekend. I do admit, the idea has appeal. We are so accustomed to expecting quick fixes for every condition that ails us that the idea of a single food or substance kick–starting the body into fat–burning mode seems almost reasonable.

Alas, many who embark on such "miracle diets" do not seem to be successful at shedding their extra pounds, especially not long term. Obesity remains a major challenge in America, where some 119 million people, or 65 percent of the adult population, are either overweight or obese (excessively fat). Excess weight is known to cause a variety of health problems, including diabetes, heart disease, cancer, hypertension, and arthritis. Being overweight is, for instance, thought to be a key risk factor for type II diabetes. In fact, a study published in the January 21, 2004, issue of the *Journal of the American Medical Association* has found that most people who are diabetic are also obese. Diabetes, in turn, increases the risk of death from several types of cancer, according to a number of studies.

Because obesity seriously predisposes people to several health conditions, it is believed to risk reversing the long-running trend toward longer life expectancy in the United States: a report published in the *New England Journal of Medicine* in 2005 predicted that life expectancy in the United States would fall dramatically in coming years because of obesity. In the following year, a study reported in the August 24, 2006, issue of the same publication showed that being obese in midlife dramatically increases the risk of dying early.

An increasingly sedentary lifestyle, too much time spent sitting in front of the TV and video game consoles, as well as wrong food choices, are also taking their toll on our children: at least 15 percent of school-age children in the United States are currently obese. In September 2006, the Institute of Medicine warned that unless urgent measures were taken, one in five children in the United States would be obese by the year 2010. The previous year, in May 2005, former president Bill Clinton and Arkansas governor Mike Huckabee were so alarmed by the prospect of America's children losing their future to overweight that they launched a campaign against childhood obesity. They announced plans to work with schools, communities, the restaurant and food industry, and the media to develop programs and policies designed to encourage healthier food choices and more physical activity.

Excessive weight is not only a national concern; it is becoming a global threat. More than one billion people—nearly one out of six—are currently affected worldwide, and the World Health Organization (WHO) has predicted that this figure could rise to 1.5 billion by 2015. No continent, and no country, is immune. In Malaysia, the number of overweight or obese people has doubled in the last decade, and there are now more fat people in Malaysia than in any other nation in Southeast Asia.

In Europe, levels of overweight and obesity are increasing at an alarming rate, with over a quarter of men and a third of women considered obese in some countries of the European Union. In Britain, where the number of prescriptions written for obesity drugs has risen by nearly 600 percent in six years, the Department of Health has warned that nearly one in three adults will be obese by 2010. A report published in October 2006 showed that Britain's adult obesity rates were the highest in Europe. Even in France, where people are reputed to have maintained healthy weight levels despite their appetite for gourmet meals and treats, waist sizes are steadily expanding. According to a 2006 survey, nearly 42 percent of the French population older than fifteen years has a weight problem. In Sweden, a recent study showed that the number of obese people had doubled in the past twenty-five years, with one in ten Swedes now considered to be overweight. In November 2006, European health experts said that Europe was facing an obesity epidemic by the end of the decade that would increase health costs and hamper economic development. Ministers and policymakers from fifty-three countries were making plans to meet in Istanbul to develop a strategy for tackling the problem and adopt a charter on countering obesity.

Developing nations, too, are increasingly affected. In India, for instance, a country where scores of people have traditionally been undernourished, there are now significant segments of the population that are overweight and obese.

Locally and globally, obesity appears to be out of control, and unless we take urgent action to contain it, we will soon have a huge runaway monster on our hands that threatens to bankrupt nations and bring our human family several steps closer to extinction.

The enormous financial weight that obesity carries is already impacting the budgets of governments worldwide. In 2003, obesity cost the United States about $75 billion, half of which was shouldered by the country's Medicare and Medicaid programs. This cost is set to increase rapidly as the medical conditions to which obesity contributes become more and more widespread among the population. Studies have estimated that annual medical expenditures for obese adults are 36 percent higher on average than for normal-weight adults. Obese patients are 3.85 times more likely to be hospitalized, and at a younger age, than nonobese patients. In 2004, Duke Medical School was setting up a course in treating obesity to provide doctors with specialized knowledge of the condition so as to be able to effectively deal with the looming obesity epidemic.

Meanwhile, treatment facilities for those with disabilities due to excess weight and obesity struggle to provide the oversized equipment necessary to do so effectively: hospitals and healthcare institutions are purchasing expensive new equipment, such as wider beds, larger blood pressure cuffs, wider wheelchairs, and reinforced toilets. Needless to say, those who lose the battle of the bulge ultimately require larger caskets when they leave this world.

At an international obesity conference in Sydney, Australia, in September 2006, Dr. Philip James, the British chairman of the International Obesity Task Force, predicted that obesity would soon "overwhelm every medical system in the world."

Malnourished heavyweights

A sad but curious paradox is that in a nation where obesity is considered to be one of the greatest threats to human health, millions of Americans don't have enough food to eat, especially nutritious food like fruits and vegetables, which are more expensive than cheaper junk foods. For some families to be able to put sufficient food on the table, it needs to be cheap, so they end up eating a nutritionally inferior meal, such as canned or packaged macaroni-and-cheese, instead of buying whole-grain pasta and unprocessed cheese and serving it with a generous helping of fresh vegetables. This way of eating promotes ill health, which necessitates medical expenses, thus perpetuating the ill-health/no-wealth cycle.

However, although obesity has long been regarded as a problem of the poor, it now increasingly affects even the more prosperous segments of the population. A recent study conducted at the University of Iowa revealed some interesting statistics: in the roughly thirty-year time span between the years 1971-1974 and 2001-2002, obesity among those making less than $25,000 per year rose 144 percent, and for those earning $40,000 to $60,000, 209 percent. When it comes to obesity, the gap between rich and poor is narrowing. But whether they are rich or poor or in between, those who carry excess weight are malnourished because they have made the wrong food and lifestyle choices.

Battle the bulge while you can

Several studies point to the importance of shedding excess weight—and keeping it off—for optimal health and enjoyment. People who are overweight in middle age, for instance, are more likely than their normal-weight peers to experience physical, emotional, and social problems when they grow old. Research conducted at Northwestern University in Chicago with nearly sixty-eight hundred overweight men and women indicates that young and middle-aged folk who carry extra pounds risk being unable to enjoy their golden years in good health. The study, published in the November 10, 2003, issue of the *Archives of Internal Medicine*, found that those who were average weight in middle age were more likely to consider themselves in excellent or very good health as they grew older. Overweight middle-aged study subjects, on the other hand, reported more frequent problems with everyday activities such as walking or climbing stairs years later. In addition, they more frequently demonstrated lower emotional well-being and impaired social functioning.

But disability due to excess weight is not limited to old age. According to a report in the January 2004 issue of *Health Affairs*, disability rates due to obesity have risen sharply over the past twenty years even among younger folk. The number of overweight people aged thirty to forty-nine who had trouble caring for themselves or performing other routine tasks increased by 50 percent during the study period from 1984 to 2000. Musculoskeletal problems, such as back problems, and diabetes were the primary reasons for the disability.

The challenge before us is clear: As individuals, families, and nations, we need to understand where we've gone wrong and take remedial action. This is neither to be found in pharmaceutical drugs, with their potentially serious side effects, nor in the increasingly popular surgical procedures, such as stomach stapling, which artificially reduces the size of the stomach, thus limiting the amount of food a patient can ingest. Instead, the answer lies in both adopting a natural whole-foods diet and increasing physical activity—a simple prescription for which we don't need a doctor, only education, understanding, and commitment. These are the prerequisites for achieving good health, and a truly healthy body will always bring its weight into balance.

Choosing a diet that fits

For those who would like to lose weight, whether it is just shedding a few stubborn pounds or a considerably larger number of them, there is no scarcity of information or advice. Just visit the health section of any bookstore or search the Internet for "weight loss," and you'll find hundreds of titles or Web sites on the topic, eagerly competing for your interest and attention. And we happily comply: on any given day, approximately one-third of the adult population in North America is on a weight–loss diet.

With so many diet plans to choose from, how can consumers know to select the one that is right for them? All types of diets have their faithful followers who will readily provide testimonials regarding a specific way of eating that finally helped them to victory in their previously unsuccessful battle of the bulge. But there are an equal number of desperate dieters who have tried it all—high and low fat; high and low protein; high and low carbs—and found that none of these diets truly made a difference for them.

By now, we've come full circle with diets advocating the consumption of considerably less or more of one of the major food categories—protein, fat, and carbohydrates. A couple of years ago, just as everyone thought the high–fat, low–carb Atkins diet had been proven the winner, a study came along suggesting that eating lots of carbohydrates, but avoiding fats, worked just as well to produce weight loss. Research reported in the January 26, 2004, issue of *Archives of Internal Medicine* concluded that a diet consisting of 60 percent carbohydrates, 20 percent protein, and 20 percent fat helped people balance their weight. Later that year, a Danish study showed that any weight loss achieved with the Atkins diet was short–lived and that after six months on the diet, people started to regain their weight.

An earlier study out of Tufts University in Boston had shown that all types of diets—from the high–fat, low–carb Atkins diet and the moderate-carb Zone diet to the extremely low–fat Ornish diet—were similarly effective in reducing weight and blood cholesterol levels. Whatever program study subjects were following, those who stayed on it for an entire year lost an average of about ten to twelve pounds, reducing their heart disease risks by 5 to 15 percent.

The major benefit for us in being offered such a varied palette of diets emphasizing different food groups is that we have become aware of the importance of quality versus quantity of food. We have begun to understand that good nutrition and weight management are not simply a matter of counting calories. Most importantly, with the introduction of the glycemic index, which is discussed later in this book, we are now recognizing that even carbohydrates are not all equal in value. New research is confirming that low–glycemic carbs, such as vegetables, fruits, nuts, and legumes, which release their sugars slowly during the digestive process, can promote weight loss, whereas high–glycemic carbs, such as refined sugars and refined grain products, which break down quickly, tend to promote weight gain.

Interestingly, the suggestion that too many starches in the diet are a major physiological component responsible for excess weight is repeatedly emphasized in the Cayce readings. These starches are said to create drosses in the system that negatively impact endocrine activity.

South Beach and Cayce

The curtailing of starches, including white rice and refined flour products such as white bread, pasta, and pastries, is also the major premise of the popular South Beach Diet. According to its creator, Arthur Agatston, M.D., South Beach is helping dieters lose between eight and thirteen pounds on average in the first two weeks.

Because eating fewer starchy foods is also strongly advocated in the Cayce readings, some have suggested that the Cayce diet and the South Beach Diet are very similar. However, the common ground of starch avoidance notwithstanding, there is an important difference between the two: The Cayce diet calls for a lot more of the "good" carbs—vegetables and fruits—than the South Beach Diet. It is based on 80 percent alkaline-forming foods, which are primarily vegetables and fruits. Meat, grains, and dairy foods, when metabolized, leave an acid residue in the body—they are thus considered to be acid-forming. For optimal metabolic function, most body fluids, including blood, need to be slightly alkaline. This improves all metabolic processes, including lymphatic function, digestion and assimilation, and immune response. The Cayce diet, therefore, emphasizes the importance of proper pH (potential hydrogen) balance, in addition to the restriction of bad carbs.

The Cayce readings also make additional recommendations—there are many finer points in the Cayce diet that are not addressed in the South Beach Diet. These include guidelines on food combining, raw foods, cooking methods, local and seasonal foods, the distinction between vegetables grown above and below the ground, and the concept that the consciousness we hold while eating, along with the thoughts we think, affects the way in which we digest and assimilate those foods. One of Cayce's most frequently quoted readings says, "What we think and what we eat—combined together—*make* what we *are*; physically and mentally." (288-38)

So, while on the surface the South Beach Diet and the Cayce diet may appear to be similar, the Cayce dietary recommendations are far more complex and detailed. The South Beach Diet prides itself on its simplicity, and it achieves results because it restricts most junk foods and refined starches, which necessarily promotes weight loss. The Cayce diet also restricts junk foods and refined starches, but it looks beyond weight loss to improved immunity and optimal protection against illness, including prevention of the common cold and serious infectious diseases. These benefits result from a healthy pH balance and optimal nutrient intake.

There are two suggestions in the South Beach Diet that I believe to be incongruent with the principles of good nutrition. One is the recommendation of low-fat dairy products. The fat in dairy is necessary because it promotes the assimilation of calcium and other nutrients. If the fat is removed, assimilation is impaired. Further, low-fat and nonfat milk products are processed with thickeners (including starches!) and additives to compensate for the loss of texture that occurs when the fat is removed. A common additive is *carrageenan*, a thickener derived from red seaweed, which in several recent studies has been shown to cause ulcerations and malignancies in the gastrointestinal tract.

My second major concern with the South Beach Diet is its liberal use of sugar substitutes and sugar-free products, which disregards the detrimental effects of these substances on the body, particularly on the nervous and endocrine systems. Sugar substitutes such as NutraSweet and Equal and products made with them contain *aspartame*, a neurotoxin reported to cause seizures; blindness; miscarriage; sexual dysfunction; obesity; and testicular, mammary, and brain tumors. In 2004, a Racketeer Influenced and Corrupt Organizations complaint was filed in a U.S. District Court against NutraSweet Co. and the American Diabetes Association for manufacturing and marketing toxic aspartame.

Among the discrepancies between the South Beach Diet and the Cayce diet is that South Beach permits pork but disallows butter. The Cayce readings advise against pork, with the exception of small amounts of crisp bacon occasionally. They do permit butter in moderation, to season cooked vegetables or as a spread on whole-grain toast. These Cayce recommendations are in alignment with current scientific findings.

At a time when obesity is a serious worldwide pandemic, we should be grateful for the South Beach Diet and other diets that are successful in helping people lose weight and thereby prevent obesity-related health problems, such as diabetes and heart disease. But as I will try to show in this book, we can confidently look to the Cayce diet as a natural, safe, and nutritionally balanced way of eating that provides all important nutrients in optimal amounts and proportions, and in that manner helps us achieve our ideal weight.

2

Give Me Five:
The Principles
of Healthy Eating

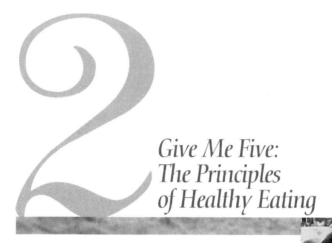

JIM DAVIS' POPULAR CARTOON CHAR-
ACTER Garfield suggests, "Never diet on
a day ending in 'y.'" I urge you to consider
the wisdom of his advice. Don't bother going
on a diet. Diets don't work, because they effectively starve an already
malnourished body. Many of the individuals who are on a weight–loss
diet on any given day will be unable to keep off the weight they may
lose, and many have already lost and regained their excess pounds
numerous times. Several studies indicate that 90 percent of those who
lose weight regain it within five years.

So, how can we turn our weight–loss resolution into a plan that works
and won't fall by the wayside? We need an emphasis on quality, not
strictly quantity, of food. Weight loss is a question of eating more of the
right foods and far less—ideally none—of the wrong foods. Some foods
clog up the digestive and lymphatic systems and thereby hinder our
efforts to shed extra pounds. Other foods promote healthy metabolic
function and thereby aid weight loss. Some foods even increase our
ability to burn fat—these are referred to as thermogenic foods.

We also know that people have different nutritional requirements based on individual biochemistry and metabolism. These are genetically predisposed, as well as influenced by past food choices, the environment we live in, the type of work we do, when and how well we sleep, and other aspects of our lifestyle. We will discuss each of these later in the book.

In the Cayce readings, the two major nutritional considerations for achieving weight loss are the recommendation to curtail starches in the diet and the suggestion to drink grape juice, diluted 2:1 with water, before each meal and before retiring at night. The readings indicate that grape juice, taken in this manner, will reduce the desire for starches and sweets, as well as balance glandular activity related to digestion. Working with these two recommendations sounds like a simple recipe for balancing weight, and anyone interested in losing weight would certainly be wise to implement them. However, considering that starches typically form such a large portion of many diets today, it is important for us to know what the best foods are to replace those starches—in other words, we need to reinvent our diet. That is why, throughout this book, we will consider the principles of a healthy diet, combining the guidelines from the readings with current scientific research. At the basis of these principles, however, is the important concept of the acid/alkaline balance.

Cayce diet 101: keeping the body alkaline

The recommendation to "keep the body alkaline" is a recurrent theme in the Edgar Cayce readings, and it is suggested that one of the ways we can achieve this is by centering the diet around alkaline–forming vegetables and fruits. We are advised that we can improve metabolic function, maintain a high state of health, and prevent colds, infections, and other illnesses by maintaining the body in an alkaline state. Reading 523–1 says, "Be mindful that the diet is such that it keeps . . . toward alkalinity for the body at all times; for this will not only prevent infectious forces but will aid in keeping the blood stream in such a manner as to aid in eliminations . . ."

Today, more than half a century after the sleeping Cayce admonished that acidic conditions predispose the body to ill health, the notion of

P. H.

pH balance is finally catching the interest of health professionals and the general public, as more and more books and various health publications focus on the issue.

The pH scale is applied to measure acidity or alkalinity of body fluids. Its values range from 0 to 14, acid to alkaline, with 7 being neutral. For optimal health and metabolic function, most body fluids must be slightly alkaline. Blood should be at or near a pH of 7.4. Whenever the scale tips, the body mobilizes a special buffering system and draws on its *alkaline reserve*, consisting of mineral stores, to neutralize acidity. However, the minerals in the alkaline reserve must be replenished regularly through food. An alkaline–forming diet is therefore important.

All foods, after being metabolized, leave either acid– or alkaline–forming elements in the body. Alkalizing foods are those which supply predominantly alkaline–forming minerals such as calcium, sodium, magnesium, potassium, iron, and manganese. Most vegetables and fruits are in this category. Acidifying foods supply predominantly acid–forming minerals like copper, iodine, phosphorus, sulfur, and silicon. Meats, grains, and most fats and dairy products belong in this group.

Many charts have been published that list foods in the acid and alkaline categories. If we consult different ones, we are likely to find numerous discrepancies, partly due to differing research criteria or to actual variations of mineral values in foods, depending on where these foods are grown and whether or not they are refined. For instance, whole grains are less acid–forming than refined grains, from which the nutrient–rich germ and bran have been stripped away. Freshly picked, sun–ripened vegetables and fruits grown in organic soil are higher in alkaline–forming minerals than those grown in chemically imbalanced soil and harvested prematurely.

The best way to achieve an 80 percent alkaline–forming diet, as recommended by Cayce, is to build our meals around fresh vegetables and fruits, with smaller proportions of cereals, dairy, and meat than are typically featured in the North American diet. Ideally, all foods should be organically grown, whole, and unrefined, so that we can benefit from the full spectrum of nutrients and thus the alkalizing potential placed in the food by Mother Nature.

Most herbs (including herbal teas), spices, and food–based nutritional supplements, such as green–food concentrates, are alkaline–forming. Freshly extracted vegetable and fruit juices are highly alkalizing. I have often witnessed someone who felt weak and exhausted perk up and feel better within half an hour of drinking a large glass of fresh vegetable juice. Hot broths made from vegetables or chicken bones, as well as miso soup, are high in alkalizing minerals and have a similar effect.

Avoid fried foods, processed foods, and foods high in refined starches and sugars, which are highly acid–forming and rob the body of nutrients when they are metabolized. Alcohol, nicotine, and pharmaceutical drugs are also acid–forming. If tolerated, a small glass of red wine per day has medicinal value, but alcoholic beverages in excess upset the body's acid–alkaline balance.

In addition to diet, lifestyle factors influence the body's pH balance. Stress, noise, environmental pollution, and lack of sleep and exercise all create acid conditions and ultimately disease. Prayer and meditation, restful sleep, and aerobic exercise such as walking, which pumps alkaline–forming oxygen into the body, are alkalizing and thus healing. Deep, abdominal breathing exercises are also recommended.

An easy way to test your pH balance is to use pH paper, or litmus paper, which is available at many health food stores and some drugstores.[1] This type of paper enables you to test the pH balance of liquids, including body fluids. To test the pH of saliva, wet the end of the paper in your mouth and, within seconds, watch the paper change its color. You will then be able to compare the color with samples shown on a color scale that indicates the matching pH level.

You can test your pH level at any time throughout the day, but you will get your most accurate values first thing in the morning. Test your values several days in a row. If your results consistently indicate a level below 6.5, you can benefit from switching to an alkaline–forming

---

[1] To order this and other Cayce products mentioned in this book, visit baar.com in the United States, and EdgarCayceCanada.com in Canada.

diet and implementing the appropriate changes in your daily routine and lifestyle.

Five principles of healthy eating

As we have seen, the Cayce dietary guidelines do not offer dogma. Rather, they show us how we can meet the nutritional needs of the physical body in the most efficient and effective way. Combining the information from the readings with current nutritional research, which increasingly substantiates Cayce, we can identify the following five principles of optimal nutrition:

1. Indulge in water.
2. Favor veggies and fruits.
3. Prioritize for protein.
4. Keep starches in check.
5. Banish fake fats.

Brief and to the point, these guidelines are easy to remember. Write them down on a piece of notepaper. Post them on your fridge; take them with you when you go to the grocery store and dine in a restaurant. Plan your meals with these principles in mind, and you'll be assured of success if your goal is greater health, abundant energy, and optimal weight.

Let's take a quick overview of each of these principles before we discuss them in greater detail in the chapters to follow.

Indulge in water. Drink six to eight glasses of filtered or spring water each day, between meals. Water is needed for the process of elimination, to flush out toxins, and to deliver nutrients to the cells. Whenever you feel hungry, drink a glass of water first, then wait fifteen minutes before you eat your meal. You'll find that you won't be as hungry, and you'll digest your food better, as you won't need to drink as much with your meal—taking liquid with meals dilutes digestive juices, thus weakening digestion.

Favor veggies and fruits. Vegetables and fruits are a storehouse of vitally important nutrients and phytochemicals that should make up the bulk of everyone's diet. Stop thinking of vegetables as a side dish on your dinner plate, and make them the center of your meals. Always include orange vegetables and dark green leafy vegetables, which are especially rich in vitamins, minerals, and antioxidants. Vegetables also supply lots of fiber, which promotes healthy bowel function. At least one–third of your veggies should be eaten raw. Raw foods supply enzymes that promote digestion and a healthy metabolism. Prepare other vegetables by steaming, baking, or cooking them in parchment paper to preserve nutrients. Eat six to seven servings of vegetables a day, more if you like. It's difficult to overeat on vegetables! Fruits are the ultimate testimony to nature's beauty and bounty. Rich in color, flavor, and aroma, they are natural superfoods, brimming with vitamins, minerals, flavonoids, and antioxidants. The soluble fiber contained in fruit helps regulate blood cholesterol and sugar levels.

There is indeed good reason why vegetables and fruits should make up the bulk of the foods we eat!

Prioritize for protein. Be sure to eat a small amount of high–quality protein two or three times each day. Many dieters make the mistake of eliminating protein foods. As a result, they become famished and weak and tend to snack frequently on carbohydrate–rich foods. Protein is required for proper metabolic function and endocrine balance. It also makes you feel satisfied and less hungry. Fish, fowl, eggs, and dairy products (ideally fermented, such as yogurt) provide excellent protein. Vegetarian sources are combinations of legumes, grains, seeds, and nuts. But remember: the protein food is the side dish on your vegetable plate— not the other way around!

Keep starches in check. Avoid starchy refined and processed foods, such as white–flour products, white rice, and refined sugar, which contribute calories but no nutrient value. Some unrefined starches, such as potatoes, and whole–grain products, such as brown rice and whole-grain bread, can be enjoyed in moderation. Most nutrition researchers today agree with the Cayce readings that it is primarily refined and starchy foods that are responsible for unwanted weight gain.

Banish fake fats. Choose the right fats for your diet. Many popular cooking fats and oils are refined, processed, and chemically altered, making them toxic and unusable for the body. Use natural fats, such as extra–virgin olive oil and butter. Natural fats promote satiety and help the body make optimal use of protein. Avoid hydrogenated fats, which are harmful to your health. Certain fats can actually encourage weight loss: omega-3 fatty acids, found in whole grains, nuts, seeds, and green leafy vegetables, boost metabolic rate and increase the body's ability to burn fat.

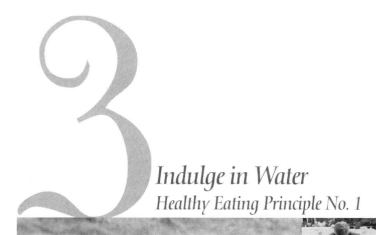

Indulge in Water
Healthy Eating Principle No. 1

THE CAYCE READINGS RECOMMEND that we "drink plenty of water through the day, at least six to eight tumblers full." (2341-1) We have all heard similar advice today—from doctors, spouses, friends, and colleagues. We listen to it and nod in agreement. But how many of us actually drink this much water every day?

Water is the most abundant substance in nature, both on our planet and in our bodies. About three-fourths of the earth's surface is covered with water. The ratio in the human body is similar—around 70 percent. It makes sense, then, that water should be considered our most important nutrient. Indeed, while we can survive without food for more than a month, we can live only a few days without water. Terri Schiavo's court-ordered death by dehydration in 2005 sadly illustrated for the world how physical functions soon shut down, one by one, when the body is deprived of water, resulting in the death of the body. We know that death by dehydration is very painful.

And while most of us are fortunate not to have to suffer this type of death, many of our everyday aches and pains are nevertheless indicative of a system–wide water shortage. Practically all metabolic processes depend on water, and if there is not enough to go around, we will begin to develop small–scale system failures, including digestive difficulties, weight gain, high blood pressure, back pain, and allergies. It may never occur to us that these problems are caused by inadequate water intake, and we may even look to pharmaceutical drugs in an effort to control symptoms that are actually water–shortage warning signals.

By dramatically increasing their water intake, many people have successfully eliminated stubborn health problems, lost weight, and gained abundant energy. Water is required for digestion and assimilation, as well as for the elimination of toxins and waste products. We depend on water to deliver nutrients to the cells and for the circulation of blood, lymph, and interstitial fluids. Water is needed for the regulation of body temperature and for the maintenance of electrolyte and osmotic pressure balance. In short, it runs the body! This is why the Cayce readings recommend that we ". . . keep the whole system, inside and out, thoroughly cleansed with water, drinking water as medicine, or in regular intervals and drinking sufficient." (4771–1)

It is best to drink most of your water between meals because drinking too much of it with meals dilutes the digestive juices, thus interfering with the digestive process. The Cayce readings advise: "Do not drink water with meals. Take the water between the [meal] periods . . ." (5647–1)

One of the recurring recommendations in the Cayce readings is that even liquids should be chewed, including water. Reading 595–1 suggests: "Even in drinking water, *chew* it—or masticate it at least three or four times. That is, sip it—let the activity of the glands in the mouth mingle well with the water; not gulping it but sipping it gently." And reading 808–3 advises, "Even milk or water should be *chewed* two to three times before taken into the stomach itself, for this makes for the proper assimilation . . . and gives more value to the whole of the body."

Increasing water intake is recommended in the readings for various conditions ranging from indigestion and general weakness to skin problems and even cancer. The readings recognize the importance of water as a cleansing agent. Reading 1586–1, given for a cancer patient, says: "First, drink plenty of water each day—six or eight glasses. It is true that this tends to flush the kidneys, and it may at times cause some inconvenience in the evening; but they must be flushed out—and water is the better to use for same, see?"

Water + walking = weight loss

Water and walking form the basis of nature's perfect weight-loss program—easy, effective, and inexpensive. The late Dr. F. Batmanghelidj made it his life's work to inform the world about the connection between inadequate water intake and various conditions of ill health, including obesity. He believed that many people who are overweight think that they are hungry, when they are, in fact, thirsty. So they reach for food instead of a glass of water. Batmanghelidj's research showed that a combination of increased water intake and daily exercise in the form of extended walks is the simple and effective answer to the problem of overweight. Drinking plenty of water before eating food satisfies the body's need for greater hydration and reduces the sensation of hunger. Through complex processes, it also provides the body with energy that would otherwise remain unrealized. Long walks, in turn, stimulate the body's fat-burning mechanism. The Cayce readings frequently advocate walking as the best form of exercise.

Dr. Batmanghelidj published several books detailing his research and experiences in helping patients overcome a wide range of health problems, with titles ranging from his classic *Your Body's Many Cries for Water* to his recently released *Obesity Cancer & Depression: Their Common Cause and Natural Cure.* Relying on simple nature cures rather than expensive pharmaceutical medication, Dr. Batmanghelidj was also the originator of the Foundation for the Simple in Medicine. Visit his Web site, www.watercure.com, for more information.

Choosing your drinking water

Now that we have established the need for drinking more water, our next question becomes, What type of water should we drink? Although, for most of us in the industrialized world, water is ubiquitous and easily accessible, we have become increasingly suspicious of pollutants and toxic residues in our water supply. Many people today choose bottled water or use filtration equipment in their homes.

Water quality appears to have been a concern even in Cayce's time, although perhaps on a lesser scale. Some of the people who received readings from Cayce asked him what water they should drink and received a very specific response. Sometimes, Cayce approved of certain brands of bottled water. In several cases, the readings suggested adding small amounts of elm, lithia, or saffron powder to water to optimize the water's cleansing and detoxification potential, or to soothe irritations in the digestive tract. A forty–two–year–old man who had a tendency to develop ulcers was told to drink . . .

> **Quantities of water! All the body would drink! Take water rather as medicine! Well that occasionally those properties in the elm or the saffron be given as an easing for the conditions in the stomach proper. Just a pinch of the elm in a glass of water—this not hot, but not ice cold. The saffron may be made into a tea, about one to twenty steeped for thirty to forty minutes, and a teaspoonful taken in half to three-quarter glass of water. These should be taken at least once each day, either or both of these.   2190-1**

Those of us looking for an ideal water source today don't have the benefit of being able to ask Edgar Cayce for advice, so we need to do our own research. If you are unsure what type of water is best for you, try to consult someone who has researched various sources in your locality. You may be able to get help from expert staff in natural food stores or in specialty stores that provide water filtration equipment.

It would make sense that mineral–rich mountain spring water with its naturally refreshing taste is the ideal water source. It is also Mother Nature's perfect alkalizer. Unfortunately, it is not accessible to many people on this planet. Most tap water and many types of bottled water are, in fact, acidic. Use litmus paper to test your drinking water, and if the results are unsatisfactory, switch your source to one that provides more alkalizing options.

If you drink bottled spring water, be sure that it is not artificially carbonated. Cayce repeatedly warned against carbonated water and other carbonated drinks, such as sodas. Some people were advised not to drink any carbonated water; others were told they could use cola drinks in moderation. Recent research has shown that carbonated drinks may raise the risk of esophageal cancer.

While heavily carbonated beverages tend to cause an accumulation of gas in the body, I have found that, on occasion, sipping a mildly carbonated water will relieve bloating and some types of stomach discomfort. Some European spring waters are naturally carbonated, meaning that their mild fizz is part of their natural makeup and has not been artificially added at the time of bottling.

Many people find that water becomes more palatable if a splash of fresh lemon or lime juice, or a combination of both, is added. I highly recommend doing this, as fresh lemon and lime help make the water more alkaline. Reading 1709-10 says that lemon juice "is a good alkalizer. Squeeze a little lime in with it also, just two or three drops in a full glass of the lemon juice taken. Best to mix the lemon juice with water, of course."

Shun sugary soft drinks

Sugary soft drinks should be avoided at all times. A report in the August 8, 2006, issue of the *American Journal of Clinical Nutrition* says that the increased consumption of sodas and sugary drinks is a key reason that more people have gained weight. The report claims that an extra can of soda per day, which delivers the equivalent of ten teaspoons of table sugar, can pile on fifteen pounds a year. Do not be fooled by so-called diet drinks, laden with artificial sweeteners and other chemicals of questionable safety. Artificial sweeteners are neurotoxins and endocrine disruptors that are known to be harmful to the body. Cola drinks also contain caffeine, which, when taken in excess, overstimulates the nervous system. However, the Cayce readings do recommend Cola syrup in small amounts, taken in plain or naturally carbonated water, for purifying the kidneys and coordinating kidney and bladder function. It also helps relieve mild stomach discomfort and upper abdominal gas.

Drinking distilled water is not recommended, because it is devoid of minerals and therefore tends to draw electrolytes and trace minerals from the body. Under professional supervision, the use of distilled water for detoxification purposes over short periods of time may be helpful, but distilled water should not be consumed on a regular basis and over extended time periods.

If you are interested in considering water energy in a totally new and different light, I invite you to study the work of the Japanese water researcher Dr. Masaru Emoto. Using high–speed photography of crystals formed in frozen water, Emoto has demonstrated that when specific, concentrated thoughts are directed toward water, the molecular structure of the crystals changes, depending on the nature of the thoughts. Loving, harmonious thoughts produce beautiful, inspiring shapes, whereas hateful, negative thoughts produce rather ugly–looking water crystals. It is as if water acts as a magnet for our individual and collective thoughts, which are then reflected back to us in the structure of the water crystals. Emoto has documented his research in his fascinating book *Messages from Water*. Photographs of several types of drinking water from around the globe demonstrate that there is indeed a world of difference between various types of water. If we don't do anything else, the least we can do is direct loving thoughts toward our water before we drink it. This can only help increase the healing potential of the water we take into our body.

4

Favor Veggies and Fruits
Healthy Eating Principle No. 2

DIETARY GUIDELINES FOR AMERICANS, which is published jointly by the Department of Health and Human Services (HHS) and the Department of Agriculture (USDA) and is updated every five years, stressed in the 2005 edition that many Americans are overweight and need to eat more vegetables, along with fruits and whole grains.

In recent years, several studies have shown that the Mediterranean diet, high in vegetables and fruits, brings many benefits to human health. This diet has been credited with increasing life span, preventing arthritis, and protecting cardiovascular health. Clearly, veggies and fruits excel in terms of the benefits they bring to our health, and they have been shown to help promote weight loss while keeping the body well nourished and the palate satisfied.

The Cayce readings recommended long ago that vegetables and fruits be at the center of the human diet, favoring especially those vegetables belonging to the green leafy, and yellow or orange, varieties. Current research has shown that these are also the types of vegetables that are highest in antioxidant properties, meaning that they are exceedingly protective of human health by preventing free radical damage in the body.

Green veggies owe their bright color to chlorophyll, an effective detoxifying and anti–inflammatory agent. Chlorophyll is also one of the best natural sources of magnesium, an important element in the utilization of calcium in the body. In addition, green vegetables supply many other minerals, vitamins, and essential fatty acids. Yellow and orange veggies are excellent sources of cancer–fighting carotenoids, as well as the B–complex vitamins and several important minerals.

It's not difficult to pack some greens into each meal. Lettuce, endive, watercress, and parsley are examples of tasty greens that provide a delicious base for a nutritious salad. The Cayce readings emphasize the purifying properties of lettuce. Reading 404–6 says: "Plenty of lettuce should always be eaten by most *every* body; for this supplies an effluvium in the blood stream itself that is a destructive force to *most* of those influences that attack the blood stream. It's a purifier." The readings stress that leaf lettuce, rather than head lettuce, should be used. With the exception of fiber, there are few nutrients in the pale leaves of iceberg lettuce. The deep green leafy varieties, such as romaine and leaf lettuce, are more nutritious, supplying calcium, magnesium, potassium, iron, vitamins B and C, and carotenoids, from which the body makes vitamin A. The coarser, darker outside leaves contain higher amounts of nutrients than the tender core leaves. But unless the lettuce is organically grown, the outside leaves have also been the target of repeated pesticide sprayings. Choose organic lettuce whenever possible.

Arugula, an aromatic salad green, is highly alkaline–forming and thereby counteracts acidic conditions in the body. It adds a mild nutty flavor to salads. Arugula supplies calcium, magnesium, potassium, and manganese, along with other important minerals and vitamins, including B complex.

Curly endive and its relative escarole add crunch and zest to salads. They are also highly nutritious, with a portfolio of nutrients similar to that of lettuce, but in higher concentrations. Curly endive and escarole are also valued for their therapeutic properties. Their slightly bitter taste benefits the liver and stimulates the flow of bile, promoting good digestion.

Dandelion greens are unjustly despised in our lawns and gardens, but we should at least learn to appreciate them in our salads. Dandelion leaves are a nutritional powerhouse, packing minerals such as calcium, iron, magnesium, and potassium, along with vitamins B, C, and E. Slightly bitter in taste, dandelion leaves have a tonic effect on the spleen, pancreas, liver, and gallbladder. By improving digestion and providing concentrated nutrients, dandelion offers healing and nourishing effects that extend to the entire body.

Watercress and parsley both have a long history of use as medicinal culinary foods. They are considered to be purifying and blood–building, providing plenty of minerals, including iron, calcium, and magnesium. Iodine, which benefits thyroid function and glandular health, is also found in watercress and parsley. Both are good sources of carotenoids and vitamin C, as well as folic acid and B vitamins. In addition, watercress supplies vanadium, which helps promote circulatory health and a strong heart. The Cayce readings recommend watercress for the treatment of anemia, arthritis, and cancer, among other conditions.

A study reported in the February 2007 issue of the *American Journal of Clinical Nutrition* showed that the regular intake of watercress offers protection against DNA damage in blood cells, considered to be an important trigger in the development of cancer. Study subjects who ate a bowlful of watercress every day for eight weeks also measured higher levels of antioxidants in the bloodstream, while triglycerides were significantly reduced.

Several Cayce readings mentioning watercress recommend that it be prepared with gelatin, which can be added to salad dressings. Gelatin acts as a catalyst, supporting optimal assimilation of nutrients from food. It also provides nutritional support to the musculoskeletal system.

Parsley is also an excellent natural diuretic and supports the healthy function of the kidneys and urinary tract. Give all your meals a flavorful nutritional boost by sprinkling them with finely chopped parsley!

No list of healthy green foods is complete without spinach, considered by many to be one of the most nutritious vegetables known.

It is a particularly rich source of cancer-fighting chlorophyll, carotenoids, vitamin C, calcium, potassium, and several B vitamins, including thiamine and folic acid. In the Cayce readings, spinach is recommended for its blood–building and –purifying properties, as well as for its ability to help soothe nervous conditions.

Prepare your green salads by chopping, slicing, or grating the ingredients. The Cayce readings suggest varying the method of preparation so as to make the greens more appealing. Reading 3564–1 advises:

> **In the matter of diet, keep plenty of raw vegetables; as water cress, celery, lettuce, carrots, mustard, onions, radishes and the like. Not necessarily all of these at any one period but some of them every day. Often prepare these with gelatin– about three times a week, for gelatin also is needed in the body. Grate them, slice them, dice them, changing their manner of preparation so as not to become objectionable.**

To add taste and aroma, olive oil, mayonnaise, or French dressings may be used. Don't be fooled by today's popular low–fat or no–fat dressings, which are hazardous to your health. Natural fats are required for the assimilation of the vitamins and minerals in green foods. A small amount of dressing goes a long way in adding zest to your salad.

You may have noticed that all the greens we have just discussed can be enjoyed in their natural, raw state—no cooking required. Indeed, this is the healthiest way to take advantage of the high nutritional boost they provide. The Cayce readings often suggest that we eat at least one entirely raw meal each day, ideally the noon meal. If that is not practical, a smaller raw salad should be taken with both the noon and evening meals.

Enzymes in raw vegetables and fruits

Eating raw foods provides the body with enzymes, which are specialized proteins present in all living cells. They are organic catalysts necessary for all physical and mental activities.

Enzymes can be divided into three major categories according to their function: metabolic enzymes, digestive enzymes, and food enzymes. Metabolic enzymes are the body's caretakers—they play an important role in cellular repair and organ function. Each body cell has numerous enzyme particles necessary for metabolic processes.

Digestive enzymes help break down food. Digestion begins in the mouth, where chewing ruptures the cell walls of the foods and enzymes are activated. (You can do a simple test of this by taking a piece of bread in your mouth and chewing it slowly. Within a few moments, you will notice a sweet taste. This is due to the action of the amalytic enzyme *ptyalin*, contained in saliva, which splits the complex polysaccharides into simple sugars.) After the food has been chewed and swallowed, it begins to be broken down by enzymes manufactured in the stomach, pancreas, and intestines. The majority of digestive enzymes are produced by the pancreas. Their release is regulated by a precise supply-on-demand process dependent on the types of foods eaten. The enzyme *amylase* digests starch, *protease* digests protein, *lipase* digests fat, and *cellulase* digests fiber. *Lactase* helps digest lactose, the milk sugar found in dairy products.

The demand for the body's digestive enzymes is greatly reduced with the intake of food enzymes, which occur naturally in all fresh and raw foods. When we eat foods in their raw, unadulterated state, the enzymes they contain are released through chewing, and they immediately activate digestion. Raw foods possess the exact amount and types of enzymes necessary for their digestion. The more raw foods we eat, the more we can help the body conserve energy for metabolic processes, including its fat-burning potential.

Think of raw foods as a deposit in your enzyme savings account. You make the deposit, and your body rewards you with interest by way of better digestion, better health, a slimmer you, and greater physical and mental energy. Up to 80 percent of the body's energy is tied up in digestion following a heavy, cooked meal. No wonder so many people feel sluggish and fatigued day after day! Include more raw foods in your diet, and you will soon feel the difference in your energy levels. You will also be surprised how much easier it is to melt off excess pounds.

Springtime and the summer months are an ideal time for increasing raw food consumption. Raw foods are cooling foods. When it's hot outside, turn off your stove and enjoy a fresh garden salad, raw veggies and dip, fresh fruit, and freshly pressed juices made from them. You will be loading your body with enzymes—a living energy that translates into greater physical and mental stamina.

Some tropical fruits are particularly high in enzymes that can assist the digestion of other foods. Pineapple, for instance, contains significant amounts of *bromelain*, and papaya is high in *papain*. Both enzymes have powerful proteolytic (protein–digesting) action. There isn't a lot of protein in pineapple or papaya, but eating these fruits with a protein-rich meal can help digest the protein in other foods.

Enzymes are destroyed by heat used in cooking. The higher the cooking temperature and the longer the process, the more enzymes are destroyed. When we eat cooked food devoid of enzymes, the pancreas must compensate for the lack by producing more digestive enzymes. To keep meeting an excessive demand caused by too many cooked foods in the diet, the pancreas will often become enlarged. Eventually, it may become exhausted and develop pathological conditions.

The long–term consumption of cooked foods thus creates a chronic enzyme deficiency, which can result in problems with digestion. Digestive complaints are one of the main reasons people visit their doctor. Once digestion is compromised, it's only a question of time before illness results.

Those who make sure to include raw foods in their diet on a regular basis find it easier to shed unwanted pounds because their digestive and metabolic power is optimized.

Cayce often suggested that raw foods be grated. An individual seeking help for endocrine imbalances was told:

> **Noons—principally (very seldom altering from these) raw vegetables or raw fruits made into a salad; not the fruits and vegetables combined, but these may be altered. Use such vegetables as cabbage (the white, of course, cut very fine), carrots, lettuce, spinach, celery, onions, tomatoes, radish; any or all of these. It is more preferable that they *all* be grated, but when grated do not allow the juices in the grating to be discarded; these should be used upon the salad**

**itself, either from the fruits or the vegetables. Preferably
use the *oil* dressings; as olive oil with paprika, or such
combinations . . .   935-1**

If it is not practical for you to increase raw food consumption, you
can still add enzymes to your diet by taking enzyme supplements.
Synthesized concentrates of plant–derived food enzymes and animal–
derived enzymes are available in natural food stores. Many people are
pleasantly surprised to find their digestive complaints, as well as
symptoms of physical and mental fatigue, disappear when they begin
taking enzyme supplements. There are many types of enzyme
supplements on the market, so be sure to obtain expert advice when
selecting the product that's right for you.

Fresh juice power

One of the best ways to add raw vegetables and enzymes to your diet
is with fresh juices. The major benefit of juicing is that it allows you to
take in high concentrations of nutrients from raw vegetables without
burdening the digestive system. Fresh juices are a great way to load up
on energy and nutrients quickly. They supply an abundance of vitamins,
minerals, antioxidants, and other phytochemicals that help protect
cellular integrity. They also promote the alkalinity of body fluids, which
is vital for proper immune and metabolic function.

A wide variety of vegetables and fruits are suitable for juicing; let
your creativity unfold as you try out different combinations. Carrot juice
and apple juice are all–time favorites that can be enjoyed on their own
or as a base to mix with other juices, such as greens, beet root, or ginger.
Potassium–rich celery is another popular flavor that combines well with
stronger tastes.

Juicing is also a terrific way to get your daily supply of greens. As we
have seen, dark green leafy vegetables such as kale, watercress, and
parsley are excellent sources of chlorophyll, vitamins, and minerals,
including easily assimilable calcium and magnesium. However, their
strong flavor can be overwhelming to the taste buds. Combining them
with milder–tasting juices makes them more palatable.

To prepare fresh vegetable juice in your own kitchen, you'll need a juice extractor. Juicers use different mechanisms for extracting the juice from the fiber of a vegetable or fruit. For everyday home use, a quality centrifugal juicer is generally the best and most economical choice. You may, however, find it useful to research the market, either via the Internet or by visiting a reputable natural food store, for the type of juicer best suited to your needs.

Now let's put our equipment to the test and juice up some great veggie combos, using organic vegetables whenever possible. As these sample recipes suggest, you can add medicinal effect to your juices by spicing them up with small amounts of add-ons such as parsley, garlic, ginger, lemon, wheatgrass, spirulina, ginseng, or cayenne.

Power-Cleansing Punch

4-5 medium-size carrots
3 ribs celery
1/4 beet root
3 sprigs watercress
1 almond-size piece ginger
1 teaspoon fresh lemon juice
Dash cayenne

Bunch up watercress and ginger and push through the juicer with carrots. Add lemon juice and cayenne.

Double Energy Delight

3-4 medium-size carrots
3 ribs celery
2 ripe tomatoes, quartered
1/4 teaspoon spirulina powder
1/4 teaspoon kelp powder

Place tomatoes in juicer first; push through with carrots and celery. Stir in spirulina and kelp.

Bio-Best Immune Booster

3-4 medium-size carrots
3 ribs celery

5 lettuce leaves (romaine or leaf lettuce)
1 apple
1 clove garlic
5 sprigs parsley
1/8 teaspoon ginseng powder
Bunch up the lettuce and parsley with the garlic, and push through your juicer with carrots, celery, and apple. Stir in the ginseng powder.

If fresh vegetable juice is not a practical option for you, you can select from a wide range of organic bottled juices, available in natural food stores. Some of these may be prepared using lactic-acid bacteria (LAB) fermentation. LAB-fermented juices have the advantage of being partially predigested through enzyme action. Starches and sugars in the vegetables have been converted into lactic acid, which eliminates putrefactive bacteria from the intestines and helps restore a healthy bowel flora, important for good digestion. LAB-fermented juices and vegetables, such as raw sauerkraut, also help the body synthesize nutrients, including choline and vitamin B12. It is important to note that a mildly acidic environment in the intestines, which is essential for keeping the growth of harmful, disease-causing bacteria in check, does not cause acidity in the rest of the body.

Ready for a juice fast?

Our bodies are continuously assaulted by toxins from pesticides in food, poisonous chemicals in air and water, prescription drugs, and toxic substances formed in the body from faulty digestion and elimination, as well as from stress chemicals. The liver is the major organ of detoxification. It works continuously to break down toxic substances, but an overload of toxins can cause this important organ to become fatigued and sluggish, and may leave you feeling that way, too. A fast of one to three days on fresh vegetable juices or vegetable broths, clear herbal tea, and lots of pure water gives the digestive system a much-needed break and the liver a chance to catch up on housecleaning. Weight loss of two or more pounds during such a juice fast is one of the beneficial side effects.

The best way to undertake a short fast is in a supportive, relaxed atmosphere, ideally supervised by a health professional, and free from stress and worry. Therapeutic massage, castor oil packs (see chapter nine), baths with ocean salts, steam baths, skin brushing, and mudpacks promote the elimination of toxins via the skin. Practicing deep breathing exercises, best enjoyed in an unpolluted outdoor environment, helps oxygenate the blood and flush out toxins. You'll be amazed at the way an effective cleansing program can make you feel lighter and more energetic again.

Following a juice fast, introduce solid foods slowly, beginning with steamed vegetables and brown rice. Then gradually return to a normal whole-foods diet as outlined in this book.

Crunchy crucifers

Broccoli, cauliflower, cabbage, collards, and kale—these humble veggies are potent nutritional medicine. Along with other members of the cruciferous family of vegetables—Brussels sprouts, kohlrabi, and mustard greens among them—they have been shown to protect against degenerative conditions, including cancer and heart disease.

Powerful phytochemicals in cruciferous vegetables, notably antioxidant isothiocyanates, are credited with regulating complex enzyme systems in the body that have the ability to arrest the growth of cancer cells. In recent years, several research studies have associated diets high in cruciferous veggies with lower cancer risk, particularly cancer of the breast, prostate, lung, and colon.

Cruciferous derives from the Latin *cruciferae*—"forming a cross." The four petals of each flower resemble a cross, and this holds true for such unlikely relatives as rutabaga, turnips, radishes, and watercress, which are also counted among the cruciferous family. With a wide range of health-boosting crucifers to choose from, it's easy to add variety to the diet while taking advantage of the anticarcinogenic effects of this special group of veggies on a regular basis.

One of today's most popular cruciferous vegetables, broccoli, was little known in North America in the first part of the twentieth century, and perhaps this is the reason it was rarely mentioned in the Cayce readings, which recommend several other crucifers as part of a healthy diet. Today, research demonstrating the anticarcinogenic properties of broccoli has undeniably established it as a health food par excellence.

Nature has packed a lot of nutrition into broccoli, which is an excellent source of vitamin C, beta-carotene, and other carotenoids. It also provides vitamin E, folate, fiber, iron, chromium, phosphorus, and plenty of assimilable calcium. The bioflavonoid quercetin, also found in broccoli, is an effective antioxidant and acts as a natural antihistamine in the body. In 2005, a study conducted at Johns Hopkins University demonstrated that compounds found in broccoli and other plant foods appear to block an enzyme that triggers inflammation in joints.

And broccoli tastes delicious! As part of a hot meal, broccoli is great in stir-fries, in soups and casseroles, or served lightly steamed on its own, sprinkled with a bit of lemon juice, sunflower seeds, or grated cheese, preferably raw and organic. Tender-crisp broccoli florets can also be served raw with a dip as a crunchy snack or appetizer. Finely chopped or grated, raw broccoli can be added to salads, soups, or other dishes.

Combining broccoli with tomatoes at the same meal appears to maximize the cancer-protective effects of both, according to a study published in the December 2004 issue of the *Journal of Nutrition*. (It is important here to note the admonition from the Cayce readings to eat tomatoes only if they have ripened on the vine, as unripe tomatoes produce toxic conditions in the body. If vine-ripe tomatoes are not available, use organic canned tomatoes without synthetic preservatives.) An earlier study showed that combining broccoli with a selenium-rich food, such as poultry, fish, eggs, nuts, mushrooms, or sunflower seeds, also increased broccoli's cancer-fighting ability.

Brussels sprouts are a flavorful winter vegetable with a nutritional profile similar to that of broccoli. Care should be taken to avoid overcooking, which causes Brussels sprouts to taste bitter. The smaller, younger sprouts are milder in flavor and can also be shredded raw into salads.

Dark green, leafy kale is another delicious crucifer that puts an abundance of nutrients on the dinner table. Kale is higher in calcium than any other vegetable. Kale and its close relative, collards, also provide iron and an abundance of carotenoids and other anti-carcinogenic substances.

All dark green cruciferous varieties, including broccoli, Brussels sprouts, collards, kale, and watercress, are high in chlorophyll, a powerful detoxifying agent that increases the vegetables' cancer-preventive effect. Calcium and magnesium, along with high concentrations of vitamins, minerals, and other antioxidant phytochemicals, are also present in a highly bioavailable form.

Cruciferous veggies should be steamed rather than boiled, or better yet, cooked in Patapar paper (parchment) to prevent loss of the nutrient-rich juices during cooking. Eating cruciferous vegetables cooked rather than raw prevents stomach bloating and gas that some people experience with their consumption. Cooking also neutralizes the thyroid-depressive effect sometimes associated with crucifers. The Cayce readings emphasize that all vegetables, including the cruciferous variety, should be cooked in their own juices, without added fats or oils, for optimal nutritional value. After cooking, they may be seasoned to taste with butter and unrefined sea salt or kelp salt.

Radishes may be grated into salads or steamed lightly. Kohlrabi, turnip, rutabaga, and cabbage are delicious in soups and stews. Cabbage can also be shredded and added to salads and stir-fries. Raw cabbage and fresh cabbage juice have been shown to protect against, and heal, stomach ulcers.

Jerusalem artichokes

The Jerusalem artichoke, a knotty, gnarled tuber which looks like a cross between a ginger root and a small potato, is not truly an artichoke, but belongs in the family of North American sunflowers. Its name is derived not from the city of Jerusalem, as one might expect, but from a corrupted form of the Italian word for sunflower, *girasole*. Because its name is often a source of confusion to the consumer, modern-day growers and food retailers have begun labeling it as *sunchoke*.

In the Cayce readings, Jerusalem artichokes are recommended as a medicinal food for several conditions, but especially for their ability to stabilize blood sugar levels. The soluble fiber *inulin* is largely responsible for this effect, which is helpful for both those with high blood sugar (hyperglycemia) and those who are prone to low blood sugar (hypoglycemia). According to the readings, diabetics who include Jerusalem artichokes in their diet on a regular basis may be able to reduce and even eliminate the need for insulin injections:

Instead of using so much insulin; this can be gradually diminished and eventually eliminated entirely if there is used in the diet one Jerusalem artichoke every other day. This should be cooked only in Patapar paper, preserving the juices and mixing with the bulk of the artichoke, seasoning this to suit the taste. The taking of the insulin is habit forming. The artichoke is not habit forming . . . 4023-1

As we have seen earlier in this book, there is a close link between type II diabetes and overweight or obesity, as the underlying dietary causes for both conditions are predominantly an excess of starchy and refined and processed foods. Consequently, low–glycemic foods that help to balance blood sugar levels, such as Jerusalem artichokes, are effectively able to improve both conditions.

Jerusalem artichokes may be prepared in a variety of ways. The raw vegetable may be grated or shredded and added to salad or cooked in the same way as a potato or added to soups, stews, and casseroles. The following reading, given for a 59-year-old woman suffering from diabetes, recommends that Jerusalem artichokes be made a part of the diet frequently and that they be enjoyed both raw and cooked, alternating their methods of preparation:

At least four meals each week should include the Jerusalem artichoke in the diet. One time this should be taken cooked, the next time raw. When cooked, prepare as you would a boiled potato; not boiled too much, but sufficient that it crumbles–and keep the juices of same in same. Hence, cook in Patapar paper . . . 2007-1

In the northern hemisphere, Jerusalem artichokes can usually be purchased fresh from November through May. They store well in the refrigerator. Dehydrated chokes in powder or tablet form are a convenient alternative during the off-season.

Nutritious sea veggies

It may surprise us to learn that some of the most nutritious vegetables grow in the oceans. Seaweeds, which play an important role in the preparation of many traditional Japanese foods, may also be among our best allies in our weight-loss program. A 2005 study conducted at Hokkaido University in Sapporo, Japan, suggests that brown seaweed, also known as *wakame*, contains a compound that promotes weight loss. According to the study, the compound, identified as fucoxanthin, induces the expression of a fat-burning protein that accumulates in fat tissue surrounding the internal organs.

Earlier studies have demonstrated seaweed to offer a protective effect against breast cancer by reducing the amount of estrogen circulating in the body. The mineral iodine, which has also been shown to play a role in the prevention of breast cancer, is also present in sea vegetables, along with other essential minerals, vitamins, and amino acids. As we have seen, iodine is of special importance for the thyroid, the master gland of the endocrine system that regulates many physiological processes and determines the rate at which the body burns fat.

Initiation into seaweed cuisine frequently requires the breakdown of a psychological barrier: many people find it difficult to accept the idea of putting seaweeds on their dinner plates. But once they have learned to prepare and enjoy these superfoods, they soon come to appreciate the special texture and full-bodied flavor that sea vegetables lend to many dishes.

Most health food stores now offer several types of dried sea vegetables, harvested in coastal regions around the world. If you are not yet familiar with sea-vegetable cookery, you may want to initially purchase the packaged varieties, which often include instructions on how to reconstitute and prepare them. The dried seaweed is usually rinsed briefly in cold water, then soaked for about ten to fifteen minutes before cooking. Be sure to allow room in the soaking dish for the seaweed to expand to up to ten times in volume. Since some of the valuable nutrients will have been dissolved in the soaking water, it is usually a good idea to retain it, either for use in the recipe itself or as a base for soups and broths.

Here's a sampling of some of the most popular types of sea vegetables:

Wakame. Tender-textured and mild-flavored, wakame adapts readily to a variety of dishes. In traditional Japanese cuisine, wakame is often added to miso soups, noodle broths, and stir-fries, or served cold as a salad with a miso dressing, sometimes in combination with sliced veggies such as cucumbers or carrots. In the family of edible seaweeds, wakame has one of the highest concentrations of easily assimilable calcium and also offers a considerable amount of protein, iron, and several trace minerals, as well as vitamins A and B, particularly niacin. Dried wakame looks crisp and almost black in color, but it quickly softens and turns deep green during the soaking process. Since it is quite tender, it should not be cooked for more than a few minutes.

Kombu. Although the dried strips of kombu appear a little stiff and can easily be broken into smaller pieces, it is seldom necessary to presoak kombu, except when specially called for in a recipe. Due to its full-bodied flavor and rich texture, kombu is ideal for use in the preparation of stews, or stock for soups and sauces. Adding some kombu to the cooking water of dried and soaked beans enhances their flavor and improves digestibility. In addition to its popular culinary uses, Japanese folk medicine values kombu for its natural diuretic properties and as a remedy for reducing high blood pressure and elevated cholesterol levels.

Nori. Nori contains more protein than any other sea vegetable. It is rich in vitamins A, B, and C, as well as a wide range of minerals. In North America, nori is usually available dried and pressed into very thin sheets, which are cut into strips and formed into the popular sushi rolls or rice balls. Smaller strips of nori can be lightly toasted and sprinkled on soups, or on tofu, rice, and vegetable dishes.

Arame and Hiziki. Mild-tasting and highly adaptable, shredded arame is often used in cold vegetable salads or cooked along with other ingredients in stir-fries and stews. Arame is usually considered the seaweed of choice when introducing someone to sea-vegetable cuisine for the first time. Although hiziki is often prepared in a similar fashion, it is coarser in texture and has a considerably stronger flavor. Both arame and hiziki are rich in calcium, but hiziki has a particularly high iron content and is valued for its blood–building and strengthening properties.

Agar-agar. Although it is manufactured from several varieties of red seaweed, agar–agar appears whitish in color and, due to its jelling ability, is often favored by vegetarians as an effective substitute for animal-derived gelatin. It is rich in fiber and a good source of several essential minerals and vitamins. Agar–agar is most commonly available in the form of flakes or bars. Using the flakes is easiest, since they require no presoaking. In macrobiotic and traditional Japanese cuisine, agar–agar is most often cooked along with fruit juice or water in the preparation of a jello, to which fresh seasonal fruit is added during the last few minutes of the cooking process. This makes for a light and easy–to–prepare dessert, which not only tastes great but is also versatile and nutritious.

Kelp. Kelp, which is valued for its high concentration of iodine, as well as the significant amounts of calcium, potassium, and iron it contains, can be purchased in powdered form and used as a seasoning, helping reduce or eliminate the need for salt. The Cayce readings recommended kelp salt as a seasoning and substitute for common table salt. Reading 1158–31 says: "To help the glandular balance better now we would use the kelp salt in the food preparations. Just used as seasoning, not as a medicine; for this carries sufficient iodines and such activity to aid the body in the present." Indeed, in naturopathic and nutritional medicine, kelp is often recommended for its ability to bring the endocrine system into proper balance. It provides nourishment for the thyroid, which controls the body's fat–burning metabolism. Kelp is also available in tablet form, for those who find its taste too strong for their palate.

Dulse. Dulse, which has a strong salty flavor, can be eaten in the dried form as a snack or added as a garnish for soups and stews. Dulse is high in iron and potassium and a good source of several essential amino acids, especially lysine. Dulse is also available in tablet form or liquid extract.

Whether you prefer your sea veggies as part of your meal or in the form of supplements, they offer a great way of adding important nutrients to your diet and enhancing your weight–loss program!

Oriental or macrobiotic cookbooks can help you with ideas on how to incorporate seaweeds into your diet.

The art of gentle cookery

Cooking always involves compromise. The high temperatures used in the process destroy enzymes and vitamins. Cooking also prompts chemical changes in food that can produce harmful substances. Heterocyclic amines, for instance, are cancer-causing chemicals created in meat from the reaction of amino acids (the building blocks of protein) and creatine (a chemical present in muscles) at high cooking temperatures. Swedish researchers recently discovered another carcinogenic chemical, acrylamide, in cooked foods, notably in starchy foods cooked, fried, or baked at very high temperatures, such as French fries, potato chips, bread, rice, and processed cereals.

As we have seen, the Cayce readings consistently stress the importance of raw foods, which hold the greatest nutritional potential and should be included in the diet every day. But cooked foods are an undeniable part of our culinary tradition and heritage. They may also have certain nutritional advantages of their own. The anticarcinogenic carotenoid *lycopene* found in tomatoes, for instance, becomes more bioavailable when it is heated in cooking or canning. And no one can deny the healing effect that a warm cup of broth or a bowl of soup brings to a chilled or tired body.

The key to healthful cooking, then, is to use methods that minimize nutrient loss and maintain the natural state of each food as much as possible.

Patapar parchment. Cooking in parchment paper is a technique borrowed from French haute cuisine (the French call it *en papillote*—"in curl paper"), which permits the cooking of foods while retaining juices. The Cayce readings recommend a stronger, reusable type of parchment— Patapar paper[2]—as the best way to cook foods. Wash and chop foods and place on a dampened sheet of parchment. Fold the corners of the

---

[2] To order this and other Cayce products mentioned in this book, visit baar.com in the United States and EdgarCayceCanada.com in Canada.

paper around the food, and tie together with a natural cotton string. Insert the pouch into a pot filled with about two inches of water, cover, and simmer at low-to-medium temperature.

This method is suitable for cooking all types of vegetables, as well as fish and fowl. It traps steam, causing food to cook in its own juices, intensifying flavor and retaining moisture and nutrients. Foods cooked in parchment require very little seasoning. After cooking, the juice that collects in the pouch should not be discarded, as it is in this liquid that many of the nutrients are dissolved. Serve the juice with the meal, or drink it separately as a nutritious vitamin-and-mineral cocktail.

Steaming. Steaming is a popular and quick method for cooking vegetables. For best results, bring water to a boil in a steamer, place chopped veggies in the steaming basket, and close the lid tightly to limit air exposure. Reduce the temperature to low. Do not oversteam; remove vegetables when they turn a bright color and are tender but still crisp. Preserve the steaming water, in which nutrients are dissolved, for use in stews, soups, or sauces; it may be frozen if not used immediately.

Nontoxic cookware. Ensure that your pots and pans are made from high-quality materials that do not allow toxic chemicals to leach into the foods during cooking. Avoid cookware made from aluminum, which tends to oxidize and combine with the foods cooked in it, particularly if the foods, such as tomatoes, release certain acids during cooking. Beware of nonstick pots and pans, since they scratch easily, allowing the coating chemicals to seep into the food. Recent research identifies these chemicals as potential carcinogens. Stainless steel, lead-free glass, and enamelware are safer choices.

Don't trust the microwave. Avoid microwaving foods, as this process has been shown to dramatically change the molecular structure of foods, in addition to destroying nutrients. Samples of cows' milk tested after exposure to microwaves showed several significant changes in quality, including increases in acidity and sedimentation, a change in the structure of fat molecules, and a reduction in folic acid content. One short-term study involving microwaved foods demonstrated that pathological changes occurred in test subjects following the consumption of foods heated in the microwave oven.

Safe cooking oils. The Cayce readings advocate cooking foods in their own juices, without adding fats or oils. After cooking, salt and butter may be added to taste.

Stir–frying, a gentler cooking method, technically takes us outside the realms of the Cayce diet, which does not recommend cooking foods in any type of oil. However, stir–frying uses lower temperatures relative to frying and deep–frying, so it is less damaging to the food. If you do wish to cook with fats or oils, use only those that remain stable at high temperatures. These are butter, extra–virgin olive oil, macadamia nut oil, and unrefined palm and coconut oil. Avoid heating polyunsaturated vegetable oils, including safflower, sunflower, and flax seed oils, as they break down quickly when exposed to air and light, causing harmful substances to develop.

Never fry or deep–fry food. The gentler methods described here can help you prepare hot meals that taste great, digest well, and support your health.

Fruits for your health

In every endorsement of healthy eating practices, fruits are mentioned alongside vegetables for their nutritional benefits and phytochemical values. Fruits are some of the most enticing and versatile foods, with a terrific potential for supporting any weight–loss program. A study reported in the July 2004 issue of the *American Journal of Clinical Nutrition* found that individuals who make long–term changes in their diet that involve boosting their intake of fruit could prevent weight gain. Daily, new studies turn up demonstrating fruit's amazing antioxidant properties.

Let's look at a few of the most popular fruits to see how they can be incorporated into the diet.

Apples. Apples are as popular as they are nutritious. In addition to being a good source of vitamins A and C, apples also provide vitamins of the B complex. They also supply considerable amounts of calcium, potassium, phosphorus, magnesium, and fiber, including pectin, which has a gentle laxative effect. A favorite fruit used in many baked desserts, apples are high in disease–fighting bioflavonoids, including quercetin, and other antioxidant phytochemicals.

Recent research has shown apples to protect against a number of conditions, including heart disease, cancer, and memory loss.

The Cayce readings frequently recommend apples, notably the "sheep–nosed" varieties, which include red and golden delicious. Most often, it is suggested that the apples be eaten stewed or baked, except when taken as part of the three–day apple diet, which was said to be a highly effective cleansing program:

> . . . occasionally—not too often—take the periods for the cleansing of the system with the use of the *Apple Diet;* that is: At least for three days—two or three days—take *nothing* except *apples–raw apples*! Of course, coffee may be taken if so desired, but no other foods but the raw apples. And then after the last meal of apples on the third day, or upon retiring on that evening following the last meal of apples, drink half a cup of Olive Oil. This will tend to cleanse the system . . .
>
> **543-26**

When shopping for apples, it is best to look for those that are organically grown. The Alar scare in the 1980s alerted us to the fact that even the apple, always considered wholesome and healthy, is commonly treated with toxic chemicals. In fact, FDA tests have detected thirty–six different pesticide residues on apples, including the fungicide captan (a carcinogen) and the insecticide chlorphyrifos (a neurotoxin). A portion of these pesticides penetrates even the flesh of the fruit and therefore can't be washed off. Remember also that nonorganic apples are heavily wax–coated to prolong shelf life. This wax, too, is not removed by washing.

Blueberries. Blueberries are the only "blue" food found in nature. They are a rich source of disease–fighting antioxidants. A recently discovered compound, pterostilbene, helps regulate blood sugar and cholesterol levels and may be a potent tool in the battle against obesity and heart disease. A study conducted in 2006 also showed that blueberry extract inhibited the growth of liver cancer cells in a laboratory setting.

Citrus fruits. Highly alkalizing and rich in vitamin C and bioflavonoids, citrus fruits and their juices (ideally freshly squeezed) promote detoxification and boost immunity. Recent research has demonstrated that citrus carotenoids may fight inflammatory disorders such as rheumatoid arthritis.

Citrus fruits are highly effective for cold prevention. Cayce reading 738-2 says, "With the cold and congestion in the present, almost an entire liquid diet would be the better—and the greater portion of it orange juice and lemon juice combined, three parts of the orange juice to one part of the lemon."

Avoid combinations of citrus fruit and grains, although a slice of whole wheat toast with citrus is acceptable. Fresh lemon juice and unpasteurized honey added to hot water are great for soothing a sore throat.

Recent research at the Scripps Clinic in San Diego showed that eating grapefruit or drinking grapefruit juice promotes weight loss. In Cayce reading 1309-4, a woman suffering from obesity who asked if she should drink orange juice, grapefruit juice, or tomato juice was told: "As we find, if taken occasionally—a small quantity of either or all of them at various times—through the day, as the activities of the body are carried on—they should be helpful to the body."

Grapes and grape juice—
nature's prescription for weight loss

It is often said that for every human ill, nature has the perfect remedy, and grapes seem to be nature's answer to those looking for help with losing weight. Highly valued for their medicinal properties all over the world, grapes are high in disease–fighting antioxidants. The Cayce readings suggest that grapes and grape juice have a toning effect on metabolism and help restore proper eliminations. In reading 2140-1, a woman suffering from faulty eliminations was told:

> **. . . have as much as the body can possibly assimilate of *grapes!* every character, or all that may be taken of the grapes, and grape *juice*. This will act as an aid in reducing those tendencies for gas. When using the juice, extract it from the fresh grapes or else use Welch's Grape Juice—but eat as much of the fresh grapes as possible to assimilate.**

Diluted grape juice (two parts juice to one part water) is recommended in the readings to help combat obesity. The grape juice is to be taken half an hour before each meal and again at bedtime until the desired weight loss is achieved. According to the readings, this will help change the way in which the body metabolizes sugars and starches, thus promoting weight loss.

A 34-year-old woman who was concerned about her weight problem asked Cayce why she had been advised to drink grape juice, to which Cayce answered, "To supply the sugars without gaining or making for greater weight." The woman then wanted to know whether the grape juice would really be effective in her weight-loss efforts. Cayce's response was clear: "If it hadn't, would it be given?" (457-8)

Fermented grape juice—wine—is recommended in several Cayce readings as a medicinal tonic. Typically, it is red wine that is said to be beneficial when taken in small amounts and combined only with dark bread. A 51-year-old woman with obese tendencies was told:

> **Wines, or such natures, may be taken more preferably *as* food; not as those that would be taken *with* food. Hence red wine—that is, Sherry or Port, or such natures—taken with sour bread, or black bread, in the late afternoon—rather than coffee or tea—is much more preferable; and it doesn't put on weight, it doesn't make for souring in the stomach— if taken in that manner; but not with other foods!**
>
> **Do these, and be patient, be consistent. And we will bring much better conditions.**   **1073-1**

For several years, researchers have been studying the health-giving phytochemicals in red wine. Several studies identified the phenolic compound *resveratrol*, found in red grapes, red grape juice, and red wine, as a potent agent in the prevention of heart disease and cancer. A report published in the December 15, 2006, issue of the journal *Cell* revealed new insight into the disease-fighting property of resveratrol, including new evidence of the compound's antiobesity action through its ability to speed up metabolism and cause muscles to burn more energy and work more efficiently. The study, conducted with laboratory mice, showed that high doses of resveratrol neutralized the ill effects of a high-fat, high-calorie diet, significantly reducing the animals' chances of becoming obese.

For students of the Cayce readings, these new findings could be the dawning of a scientific explanation and confirmation of Cayce's claim of the weight-loss-inducing properties of grape juice. Quite likely, however, the scientists behind this research would say that the small amount of grape juice or wine recommended in the readings could not possibly supply enough resveratrol to produce the effects observed in the laboratory studies. Yet the readings even recommend that the grape juice be diluted!

In this context, I invite you to consider the homeopathic principles according to which the energetic effect of a substance becomes more potent in dilution. It may play a role here, or there may be other factors involved that have not yet been discovered or considered. The information offered in the Cayce readings has long been decades ahead of its time. Science is catching up and exploring new dimensions, but others remain untapped. What is exciting to observe is that in the case of grapes, grape juice, and wine, as in so many other fields of research, the Cayce readings and modern science are standing on common ground.

In the following pages, I have outlined some of the ways in which vegetables and fruits are best stored and preserved. I believe that it is important to know all we can about vegetables and fruits and how we can truly maximize their presence in our daily diet. Although farm-fresh, never-frozen-or-canned foods are always best, having the option of canned or frozen produce may be the only way that some of us will ever get the amount of vegetables recommended in the Cayce diet. And, as we will see shortly, eating canned or frozen vegetables and fruits is better than not eating any.

At the end of the chapter, we will also look at organic foods and why it is important for consumers to shift from being customers of large-scale commercial agriculture, which relies heavily on pesticides, to supporting a healthier, non-toxic way of growing food. But here again, if your options are limited, then commercial vegetables and fruits are better than none. It is important that you know your options, so you can aim to make informed choices.

Keeping your veggies and fruits fresh

Freshness! We all want it from the foods we eat. "Fresh," say the tags on fruit and vegetable bins in the grocery store. But how long does fresh food stay fresh?

Unfortunately, any type of storage results in some deterioration. Produce on store shelves has already begun to lose vitamins, and nutrient losses multiply each day. Wilting is a sure sign of nutrient loss, especially of climate–sensitive vitamin C. Lettuce, kale, chard, and other leafy greens that are prone to wilting register a higher ascorbic acid reduction after several days of optimal cold storage than does cabbage, which is more resistant to wilting. Green beans lose 58 per cent of their original ascorbic acid during the first three days of refrigeration after harvesting.

While a certain amount of nutrient loss is inevitable, we can minimize it by purchasing the freshest possible produce and storing it under optimal conditions.

Refrigerate all leafy greens, such as lettuce, dandelion, collards, mustard greens, chard, watercress, and broccoli as soon as possible after buying. Discard bruised and damaged leaves and keep all greens wrapped in plastic to prevent loss of moisture and vitamins. Leafy greens stay fresh only a few days. Cabbage, a popular winter vegetable, keeps for several weeks. Cucumbers and eggplant are best stored in paper bags in the crisper to protect against excessively cold temperatures, which cause the formation of pitted, mushy spots.

Refrigerate carrots or store in a cool place in perforated bags or containers to allow air circulation. This prevents the formation of terpenoids, which give carrots a bitter taste. Protected from heat and light, carrots retain their nutrients for up to seven months. Their beta carotene content actually increases during the first five months of storage, then remains stable for two months before decreasing. If you purchase carrots whose green tops are still attached, be sure to remove these before refrigerating the carrots. If you leave the greens attached, they will continue to draw nutrients from the carrot roots, which will become soft and wilted.

Potatoes are ideally stored in a root cellar or a dark, dry, and cool cupboard to prevent sprouting and mold growth. They will keep for several weeks. Potatoes stored too warm will develop dark spots and wilted skins. Potatoes that have been refrigerated turn dark more quickly after cooking. Taking them out of the fridge several hours before cooking can prevent this. Store winter squash in the same way. Tomatoes tend to lose flavor if refrigerated. They are best stored loosely in a basket that permits air to circulate. Unripe tomatoes should be stored on a counter or on top of the fridge, which allows the ripening process to continue. Remember, however, that the Cayce readings advise against consuming tomatoes that have not been vine-ripened—see the information on canned tomatoes in the upcoming section on preserving vegetables and fruits. Unfortunately, it is becoming quite difficult to find vine-ripened tomatoes nowadays.

Keep apples refrigerated to prevent spoilage and loss of moisture. In this way, apples can be stored for several months, but gradual loss of nutrients, especially vitamin C, still occurs with lengthy storage. Store apples away from vegetables, or keep them in a plastic bag, as they give off ethylene gas as they ripen, promoting spoilage of other produce.

Most pears, unfortunately, are sold unripe and must be allowed to ripen at room temperature for several days. Later, store them in the fridge in perforated bags or containers. Depending on the variety, pears can be stored under refrigeration from one to three months, during which time a gradual nutrient loss occurs.

Oranges, grapefruit, and lemons may be stored at room temperature for several days. They will last up to two months if refrigerated. Ripe peaches and plums will keep in the fridge for about a week. If they are not ripe when you buy them, store them in a brown paper bag at room temperature for two to three days, then refrigerate.

In a busy world where few folk have the time to shop for produce daily, let alone grow their own food, we need to maximize storage options so we can derive optimal freshness and nutrition from all our fruits and veggies.

Preserving vegetables and fruits: canning, freezing, drying, and fermenting

Our ancestors invested considerable time and effort in preserving food for the winter months by canning, drying, and fermenting the fruits of the harvest. Today, few households still do their own preserving, and most of it is done by commercial food processors, whose products we later purchase in cans, jars, or plastic packages. Modern refrigeration techniques have also added freezing to the variety of food-preserving methods.

What are the relative merits of the different methods, and how do they affect the nutritional value of our food? Let's take a closer look.

Canning. The canning process involves placing food in jars and heating them to high temperatures in order to destroy microorganisms that could cause the food to spoil. The jars are then vacuum-sealed, preventing air and new microorganisms from entering. When done properly, canning is a safe, time-proven method for preserving harvest-ripe food without the need for additives or preservatives.

Canned food does have a drawback, however: it is devoid of enzymes. Enzymes, which are naturally present in fresh and raw foods, are required for digestion and for all metabolic functions in the body. Enzymes are destroyed when foods are heated above 118°F. The rate of destruction accelerates with increased temperatures and longer cooking time. Temperatures used for home-canning range between 210°F and 240°F, higher for commercial canning. If enzymes are not taken in with food, the body must produce its own digestive enzymes. The long-term consumption of enzyme-deficient foods can exhaust the organs of digestion and lead to various health problems, including chronic degenerative disease. If you frequently eat canned food, be sure to take a good enzyme supplement, available in health food stores.

How does canning affect vitamins and minerals? According to research conducted by the University of Illinois Department of Food Science and Nutrition, vitamin and mineral levels in commercial canned foods are relatively stable and comparable to those of fresh foods. However, the research does not distinguish between naturally present nutrients and those that are added in the canning process. For instance, canning companies add calcium chloride to canned tomato pieces to keep them firm. Vitamin C is often added to canned fruit to maintain color. Much of the fruit's own vitamin C content is destroyed by heating. Canning also reduces B vitamins, notably folic acid, which is especially important to women of childbearing age. Vitamins A, D, and E, as well as minerals, are more stable in canned foods.

In the few references that were made to canned foods in the Cayce readings, the concern was expressed that fruits or vegetables be preserved in their own juices and without the use of sodium benzoate as a preservative. Reading 2084–1 says: ". . . [in the diet, have] rather the fresher variety [of vegetables]. However, those that are canned without Benzoate of Soda as a preservative may be taken through such seasons or periods when these are not obtainable fresh."

In the case of tomatoes, which were said to be highly nutritious when ripe, the readings emphasized that, unless vine–ripened tomatoes were available locally, canned tomatoes were, in fact, the better choice.

A middle–aged man who quite obviously loved tomatoes asked Cayce:

(Q) What has been the effect on my system of eating so many tomatoes?
(A) Quite a dissertation might be given as to the effect of tomatoes upon the human system. Of all the vegetables, tomatoes carry most of the vitamins in a well-balanced assimilative manner for the activities in the system. Yet if these are not cared for properly, they may become very destructive to a physical organism; that is, if they ripen after being pulled, or if there is the contamination with other influences . . .

The tomato is one vegetable that in most instances (because of the greater uniform activity) is preferable to be eaten after being canned, for it is then much more uniform.

584-5

Freezing. This popular method is one of the simplest ways to preserve foods at home. Both fresh and cooked foods can be preserved quickly, with minimum effort and time. Use rigid containers or flexible bags or wrappings that are moisture-resistant and leakproof. It is not necessary to sterilize foods first, as freezing significantly slows down enzymatic changes in the food that would normally cause spoilage. However, commercial frozen foods are often blanched (scalded) prior to freezing, causing enzymes and vitamin C to be destroyed.

The vitamin and mineral content of unblanched frozen foods is relatively stable. However, some nutrition experts are concerned about the destructive effect of molecular expansion that occurs with freezing, causing the cells to burst and leaving frozen produce mushy and limp when thawed.

When asked how frozen foods compared with fresh and if freezing destroys vitamins, the sleeping Cayce answered:

> **This would necessitate making a special list. For, some are affected more than others. So far as fruits are concerned, these do not lose much of the vitamin content. Yet some of these are affected by the freezing. Vegetables—much of the vitamin content of these is taken, unless there is the re-enforcement in same when these are either prepared for food or when frozen.   461-14**

It is not clear what the "re-enforcement" might be that this reading refers to. It is likely that since Cayce's time, there has been considerable improvement in the technology used for freezing foods. Most experts agree that foods which are flash-frozen immediately after picking tend to retain more nutrients than foods that are stored for several days after picking. One thing is absolutely certain: frozen veggies are far better than no veggies, and they are definitely preferable to wilted veggies.

Drying.   Drying is one of the oldest methods of food preservation. Almost any type of food can be dried, but the most popular is fruit, which makes a nutritious, tasty, quick-energy snack when dried. Foods can be sun-dried or oven-dried, but best results are achieved with a dehydrator specially designed for this purpose.

Drying concentrates the nutrient content of food. Many dried fruits are excellent sources of iron, potassium, and magnesium. Remember, however, that any pesticides and preservatives present in the fresh food will be concentrated in the dried version, so be sure to use organic produce for drying, and buy only organic dried foods. Nonorganic dried fruits are also often preserved with sulfur dioxide to maintain the fruit's bright color and "fresh" appearance. Sulfur dioxide can cause serious allergic reactions in some people. It also destroys B vitamins in the body and has been linked to kidney malfunction.

Fermenting. Before the advent of refrigeration, people relied on fermentation with lactic acid bacteria (LAB) to prevent spoilage. Fermented foods are again popular today, as information about the considerable health benefits of LAB is coming to light. LAB are natural residents in the human intestinal tract. They promote the assimilation of nutrients in the body, particularly the synthesis of B-complex vitamins and calcium. LAB have been shown to be effective in reducing serum cholesterol levels and lowering the risk of bowel cancer. The regular ingestion of sauerkraut and other LAB-fermented vegetables helps recolonize the intestinal mucosa with beneficial bacteria.

Almost any vegetable can be fermented, but the most popular ones are cabbage, radish, carrot, and beet. Sauerkraut, for instance, can be made at home by mashing shredded raw cabbage to squeeze out the juice, mixing the pulp and juice with unrefined sea salt and purified water, then packing it all tightly in a Mason canning jar and allowing it to stand at room temperature for several days. The naturally present LAB then initiate the fermentation process, which converts the sugars and starches in the cabbage into lactic acid.

When purchasing commercial sauerkraut and other fermented veggies, be sure to choose a raw, unpasteurized product, found in the refrigerated section of natural food stores. Avoid canned, pasteurized versions. The heat used in pasteurization to extend shelf life destroys enzymes and beneficial microorganisms. Unpasteurized LAB-fermented vegetables are living foods that are naturally preserved and will keep fresh in the refrigerator for several months in an unopened package, and at least one month if stored in a closed container after opening.

Locally grown and seasonal foods

If we preserve our own foods, we have greater control over the locality in which they are grown—we can rely on foods that are locally cultivated and harvested. The Cayce readings advocate the consumption of local foods, suggesting that "shipped vegetables are never very good." (2-14) Foods grown in the vicinity of where a person lives, the readings say, help acclimatize the body and align its energies with those of our environment.

Aside from such intriguing metaphysical considerations, transporting foods over long distances and across continents compromises their nutrient value. It also produces environmental concerns in terms of fuels and packaging used for transportation. The closer we stay to the home front in sourcing our vegetables, the better it is for us and our relationship with our food and our environment.

When we do this, we are also more likely to rely on seasonal foods, which are perfectly designed by Mother Nature to provide us with the exact nourishment our bodies require at specific times of the year. By building our diet around seasonal foods, we live in harmony with nature's rhythms and our environment. Traditional medical systems around the world, such as Chinese medicine and Indian Ayurvedic medicine, have long emphasized the importance of living and eating with the seasons and in harmony with our local environments.

Above and below ground

An unusual food-combining guideline from the Cayce readings calls for balancing each vegetable grown below the ground with at least two or three above-ground vegetables. Reading 677-2 says:

> **. . . a well-balanced vegetable diet, with three vegetables grown above the ground to one grown below; though such vegetables as turnips, parsnips, beets, carrots or radishes may be included among those grown above the ground— that may be used either raw or cooked as the regular vegetables. But either Irish or sweet potatoes, or rutabaga (turnips and rutabaga will be different for this body!) are those vegetables to be warned of.**

Specific energetic qualities of above- and below-ground vegetables notwithstanding, the root vegetables for which the readings seem to have issued quantity restrictions feature a high starch content. Remember that excess starches were identified in the readings (and by modern science, as we will see shortly) to be a major contributor to weight gain.

For above- and below-ground vegetables and local and seasonal produce alike, we would be wise to consider organic choices for our fruits and veggies.

Why eat organic?

Organic fruits and vegetables are grown without the use of pesticides, fungicides, and synthetic fertilizers. Organic produce is naturally healthy. Why? Think of a person who has built up a strong immunity to viruses and bacteria using good nutrition, exercise, and a healthy lifestyle. Such a person does not need pharmaceutical drugs, antibiotics, or immunization. This is the natural state of good health in humans! Similarly, crops grown in fertile, mineral-rich soil are strong and pest-resistant. They do not need pesticides, fungicides, and fumigants. This is the natural state of good health in organic fruits and vegetables!

One of the methods used by organic farmers to achieve soil health is continuous crop rotation. By moving crops to different soil patches each growing season, the organic farmer encourages soil regeneration and prevents the depletion of specific nutrients. Conventional farming methods often compromise soil health by relying on monoculture farming, which means that the same crops are planted in the same soil year after year. This seriously reduces the levels of vital nutrients in the soil and ultimately causes erosion.

Synthetic fertilizers, too, disrupt soil balance and upset the delicate ecosystem. Nitrogen fertilizers, for instance, stimulate heavy weed growth, which in turn prompts greater pesticide use. Nitrogen fertilizers also contaminate the groundwater with nitrates. In addition, they distort the crops' nutrient profile by encouraging excessive water uptake. While this causes the crops to grow quite large, it also effects a dilution of nutrients due to the higher water content. The consumer pays for the greater weight, but gets fewer nutrients per weight unit.

Soil fertilization on organic farms is accomplished with composted organic materials, including manure and nutrient-rich sea kelp. Most or all of the organic manure is produced on the farm itself, rather than being purchased elsewhere. This encourages a self–sufficient, ecologically responsible farming system that reduces waste and keeps resources on the farm.

Organic farmers also rely on other natural methods, such as companion planting, mulching, and weeding, to maintain soil and plant health. Any pest problems that do arise are controlled with organic remedies, such as biodegradable botanical soaps, sprays, and other ecological methods that work *with* nature rather than against it. Organic farming does not permit the use of irrigation with sewage sludge, the irradiation of plants or seeds to kill bacteria, or the use of genetically engineered plants, seeds, or fertilizer compounds.

Organically farmed livestock is raised in a humane manner in natural surroundings that attempt to duplicate the animals' natural habitat. Herd sizes are kept small to facilitate healthy interactions between farmworkers and animals in a caring environment. The animals are allowed ample access to pasture, weather permitting. All feed must be organic, and pharmaceutical drugs are replaced by homeopathic medicine and other natural remedies as much as possible. The routine administration of growth hormones and antibiotic drugs is not permitted on organic farms.

Is organic food more nutritious?   Common sense tells us that fruits and vegetables grown without synthetic chemicals in naturally cultivated soil are better for our health than those dowsed with pesticides and other toxic substances. A number of recent studies have also demonstrated the nutritional superiority of organically grown produce. Studies conducted in 2001 in France and the United Kingdom concluded that organic produce averaged higher levels of vitamins A, B, C, and E, and the minerals zinc and calcium, along with other beneficial phytonutrients. Research reported by the American Chemical Society in June 2002 found that organic oranges, for instance, contained 30 percent more vitamin C than their conventional counterparts.

Response from the public is clear: According to the Organic Trade Association, organic food sales in the United States grew consistently at annual rates of 15 to 21 percent since 1997, reaching $13.8 billion in consumer sales nationwide in 2005. The growing organic wave has also hit mainstream grocers, who have responded by setting up special organic sections in produce departments nationwide. Demand, in fact, has grown so much that it frequently exceeds supply.

The organic movement is also well established in Europe, where a recent opinion poll revealed that 72 percent of Europeans support organic food production. As well, a twenty-year study conducted by Swiss scientists, published in 2002, offers a strong endorsement of organic farming methods.

Britain is the world leader in organic food sales, with sales climbing 25 percent annually. Here, organic foods are not just found on private dining tables: Bronllys Hospital in Powys recently began serving organic milk to patients and staff, in response to government research showing that traces of the toxic pesticide lindane had been found in conventional milk. Lindane has been linked to cancer and to hormone disruption in humans.

In the United States, too, hospitals are increasingly looking to find ways to offer patients meals made with organic ingredients. They have begun to recognize and honor the connection between human health and our environment, as well as food and patient health.

Personal and planetary health. We might think that a switch to organic foods is a strictly personal choice, but we would be ignoring the larger picture. Pesticide-based agricultural practices are a threat to everyone's health because they undermine the well-being and ecology of the planet that sustains us. Worldwide, several billion pounds of pesticides are applied every year. Direct and indirect exposure to pesticides (in farmworkers and their families, for example) has been linked to various forms of neurological and degenerative disease.

Topsoil erosion has reached pandemic proportions. And many of the synthetic fertilizers used in intensive farming are highly soluble and readily enter ground and surface water. Thousands of tons of nitrogen fertilizer applied by conventional agriculture are not removed with the harvest each year. Think about it. If we do not stop this madness, what will happen to our water supplies?

We saw earlier in this chapter that apples are among the fruits most heavily treated with pesticides. It may be surprising that several others of our favorite fruits and vegetables are also among this group. Here is a partial list

Bananas. Pesticides used on banana plantations include chlorphyrifos and the chemical benomyl, which has been linked to birth defects. In Costa Rica, a major exporter of bananas, 35 percent of the country's pesticide imports are applied to bananas. As if pesticides were not enough, bananas are also artificially ripened with ethylene gas.

Grains. Who would think that wholesome staple foods such as grains, including rice and oats, have some of the highest levels of pesticide residues? Rice is contaminated both by the pesticides that are applied to the crops themselves and by water–soluble insecticides and fungicides that have seeped into the groundwater near rice fields. Both imported and domestic types of rice are affected. Oats and other popular grains are subject to similar contamination.

Green beans. Neurotoxins and endocrine–disruptor chemicals are among the chemicals applied in the process of growing green beans. In total, there are sixty different pesticides registered with the Environmental Protection Agency for use on green beans. Of particular concern are green beans imported from Mexico; many of these crops are contaminated with illegal pesticides.

Peaches. Like the apple, this popular fruit is subject to repeated pesticide applications. According to a report by the Environmental Working Group (EWG; www.ewg.org), a non–profit environmental organization based in Washington, D.C., peaches, apples, and nectarines are the most common source of exposure for young children to unsafe levels of organophosphate pesticides. The next time you give your little one a juicy peach, make sure it is organic!

Strawberries. Everyone knows that strawberries are a seasonal fruit, yet they are now available almost year–round. But we pay a high price for this luxury. An EWG study considers strawberries to be the single most heavily contaminated fruit or vegetable. Strawberries are also the target of genetic engineering. For instance, some of the genes from strawberries that are available out of season may have been spliced with cold–water fish genes in an attempt to make the strawberries more resistant to frost.

Why pay more for organics? Why do organic foods have higher price tags? Is it fair that we are paying a premium for natural foods?

Perhaps we need to turn these questions around: Is it fair that farmers using intensive chemical agricultural practices enjoy tax breaks and indirect subsidies, such as public and private research dollars, for growing foods dowsed with toxic pesticides? Considering the "hidden" costs to personal health and the environment, such as soil, air, and water contamination; loss of biodiversity; soil erosion; and the resulting medical expenses—are non-organic foods really less expensive?

Organic farms typically operate on a small scale, which means that organic farming is considerably more labor-intensive. The avoidance of chemicals also translates into more hours of labor in terms of tending the fields through manual weeding and other time-consuming tasks. Organic farmers and processors must pay for the cost of organic certification, which requires documentation of all the steps involved in organic production—from soil management and seed purchase to harvesting, handling, and shipping. None of these costs are subsidized by chemical and pharmaceutical manufacturing giants, so they must be added to the price of the product.

However, when we consider the impact of agricultural chemicals on our health, the health of Planet Earth, and the health of our children and future generations, it becomes clear that none of us can afford not to buy organic!

Clearly, conventional agriculture is hazardous to human and environmental health. As consumers, we have the power to register our vote in favor of organic farming each time we shop for groceries. In our role as stewards of Planet Earth, we must embrace and support the natural ways of food production that will not only put food on our table but also on the tables of our children and those of future generations.

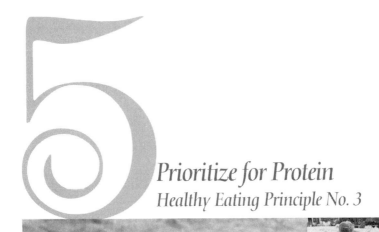

Prioritize for Protein
Healthy Eating Principle No. 3

A STUDY PUBLISHED in the July 2005 issue of the *American Journal of Clinical Nutrition* suggests that the popular low-carbohydrate diets appear to be effective for weight loss because they force people to eat more protein. According to the researchers, the increased protein intake serves to suppress dieters' appetites and thus causes them to consume fewer calories.

The word *protein* is derived from the Greek *proteios*, which means "of first importance" and reflects the undisputable importance of protein in human nutrition. Proteins are composed of amino acids, most of which the body is able to manufacture from a variety of raw materials. There are, however, at least eight essential amino acids that must be obtained from the diet. All foods, including vegetables and fruits, contain some amino acids, but the ideal ratio of the eight essential ones is present only in meat, fowl, fish, eggs, and dairy products. By properly combining certain plant foods, such as grains and legumes, nuts or seeds, that complement each other's amino–acid profile, it is possible to obtain complete protein even from a plant–based diet, although some individuals do not have the digestive capacity to do so effectively. Protein stimulates the production of the hormone glucagon, which enables the body to burn off stored fat. It is therefore important in any weight–loss program. The Cayce readings recommend fish, fowl, and lamb, as well as other protein foods, such as eggs and dairy, to be taken in moderate quantities. Once again, let us remember that protein's role is to be a side dish on your vegetable plate. Any "vacancy" created by the absence of refined carbohydrates is best filled with nonstarchy vegetables and fruits.

Meat and fish should never be fried, but rather roasted, baked, or broiled. Eating red meat is not generally recommended. A study published in 2005 found that high consumption of red meat over a long period of time could raise the risk of developing colorectal cancer. In an earlier study, researchers had found that a high level of red meat consumption could also be a risk factor in developing inflammatory arthritis.

The Cayce readings suggest that the best way to benefit from red meat is to take small amounts of juice extracted from it through heat. Beef juice, in particular, is considered to have medicinal value and is especially recommended for its strengthening properties for those who are ill or convalescing. Pork is generally advised against in the readings.

Wild game, on the other hand, including rabbit and squirrel meats, as well as organ meats such as liver, kidney, and brain, are occasionally recommended for their nerve– and blood–building properties.

The important point to remain aware of is that protein foods are essential, but only required in relatively small quantities.

Now let's review some of our best protein sources in detail.

A fresh look at whole eggs

Who's afraid of eggs? Should we be? We've often been told that eggs cause high blood cholesterol, weight gain, and heart disease. Consequently, many of us have cut eggs from our diet and use processed egg substitutes instead. If we dare eat eggs at all, we restrict our consumption to egg whites.

It's time to take another look. The natural, whole, fresh egg, and especially the yolk, is one of the healthiest and most nutritious foods around. The Cayce readings frequently recommend eggs, preferably soft–boiled or poached, and often for the breakfast meal. Conditions for which egg consumption is advised include anemia, skin disorders, and general debilitation. Most often, the readings suggest that only the yolk be eaten, since egg whites are difficult to digest.

Eggs, particularly those from pasture–fed hens or hens fed flax or fish meal, are an excellent source of balanced protein; vitamins A, B, D, and E; calcium; phosphorus; iron; and essential fatty acids. The yolk also provides lecithin, a phospholipid that promotes the synthesis of cholesterol. A substance often misunderstood today, cholesterol is a disease–fighting antioxidant and a precursor to important hormones, bile salts, and vitamin D. Research has shown that dietary intake of cholesterol has little or no effect on cholesterol circulating in the blood. High serum cholesterol is not the cause of heart disease, but rather one of its indicators, since cholesterol is a repair substance that helps heal arterial damage. Many experts even disagree with the theory that high cholesterol levels are indicative of a health problem, since several studies have shown that high cholesterol is not a risk factor for coronary heart disease. We need not fear egg yolks, or other sources of dietary cholesterol, unless the cholesterol is oxidized through exposure to air and excessive heat, such as occurs when eggs are dried and powdered. Oxidation damages cholesterol and makes it toxic to the body.

Research conducted at Yale University in 2005 showed that eating eggs every day does not increase LDL (bad) blood cholesterol or the risk for heart disease. In fact, in study participants who ate two eggs per day for six weeks, both LDL and total blood cholesterol levels did not increase and the functioning of the arteries was not impaired. Researchers concluded that there is no need for restricting egg intake in healthy individuals.

Two recent studies have also identified eggs as being potential weight–loss facilitators. Research conducted in 2004 by the Department of Food Science and Human Nutrition, University of Illinois at Urbana–Champaign, showed that the consumption of high–quality protein, such as the protein found in eggs, notably the amino acid leucine, helps reduce loss of muscle tissue, promote loss of body fat, and stabilize blood sugar levels. And a 2005 study reported in the *Journal of the*

American College of Nutrition (Vol. 24, No. 6, 510–515) showed that eating eggs for breakfast can reduce hunger and caloric intake both at lunchtime and over the subsequent twenty-four hours. The researchers believe that this may be due to the feeling of satiety that eggs provide.

Why, then, would we forgo a wholesome, nutrient–dense food such as the egg for processed substitutes, some of which are made with pasteurized egg whites and contain artificial colors, flavors, and texturizers to make the product look and taste like eggs? Other "egg replacers" contain no egg substance at all, but are made with ingredients such as vegetable protein; corn, wheat, or potato starch; soy flour; tapioca flour; carbohydrate gum; leavening agents; and various preservatives–all substances whose nutritional value is substantially inferior to that of whole eggs.

When shopping for eggs, be sure your choice is organic, or at least free–range, flax–fed, and from hens that have not been given antibiotics and other additives in their feed.

Store your eggs in the fridge in their original container, with the small end facing down. This allows the yolk to become submerged in the egg white, which protects the yolk through its antibacterial properties. Do not wash eggs before storing. This would destroy their natural protective coating and make the eggshell more porous and susceptible to penetration by harmful microorganisms. For optimal freshness, consume eggs within two to three weeks of purchase. To check eggs for freshness, place them in a bowl filled with cold water. Eggs that are old will float to the top and should be discarded.

Milk in the making

Most of the milk we are able to buy today is processed. Unless we are privileged to own dairy cattle, we usually cannot obtain unprocessed milk. Commercial milk, whether organic or not, is pasteurized, meaning it has been heated to very high temperatures to kill bacteria and extend shelf life. The heating process also destroys enzymes naturally present in raw milk that would normally assist in the digestion of the milk. No wonder many people have digestive complaints following the consumption of dairy!

Pasteurization also destroys vitamins B and C in milk and makes all remaining nutrients, including calcium, less bioavailable. In addition, most commercial milk is homogenized, which means that the fat droplets are emulsified to prevent the cream from separating.

Even in Cayce's time, pasteurization was a concern, as the following reading indicates:

> **Raw milk, to be sure, is better—but pasteurized milk needs to have that added that will make for a better activity with the gastric juices, under the disorders as have been existent in the system. Those like the Bulgarian forces, as make for the proper reaction of the bacilli that becomes active with the gastric juices.**   **404-2**

"The Bulgarian forces" are the bacteria present in fermented milk products, such as buttermilk or yogurt. It is, in fact, possible to "undo" some of the damage of pasteurization, and add a degree of wholeness back into dairy products, through fermentation with lactic acid bacteria. These "friendly" bacteria predigest the protein, fat, and milk sugar, so that the milk becomes easier to digest and assimilate. Yogurt, kefir, buttermilk, and sour cream are popular dairy products that have been made more bioavailable through the activity of bacterial culture.

Yogurt may also help you to lose weight. A study published in the April 2005 issue of the *International Journal of Obesity* showed that dieters who ate three daily servings of yogurt lost more abdominal inches and fat tissue than those who did not. In 2006, researchers at Washington University's Center for Genome Sciences also discovered a link between gut bacteria and obesity.

Buy only certified organic dairy products, made from milk given by healthy cows raised without growth hormones and antibiotics. Look for yogurt made from non–homogenized milk in your health food store. Always choose whole, full-fat milk products, and stay away from low-fat and skim milks. The fat naturally present in whole milk is required for the absorption of the fat–soluble vitamins A, D, and E, as well as for the assimilation of calcium and other nutrients. Powdered skim milk, which contains harmful oxidized cholesterol, is added to 1 percent and 2 percent milk. Avoid low-fat yogurt and sour cream, which often contain mucopolysaccharide slime or other unhealthy substances to give them body and texture.

Many traditional European cheeses, as well as certain organic cheeses made in Quebec, Canada, are made from enzyme-rich raw milk, which makes them easier to digest than cheeses produced from pasteurized milk. In contrast, the popular even-textured processed cheeses and cheese spreads contain emulsifiers, extenders, colorings, phosphates, hydrogenated oils, and other undesirable additives. These are hi-tech "plastic" foods that should be strictly avoided by health-conscious consumers.

The Cayce readings recommend that cheeses be eaten in moderation, and soft types of cheese are preferred. Eating cheese at the same meal as other protein foods, or combining cheese with quantities of starches, is advised against. Quantities of high-protein and high-starch foods should not be combined in the same meal because protein and starches require different gastric secretions for their respective digestion.

Storing milk and cheese. Until pasteurization became mandatory, it was unnecessary to refrigerate milk. Left to stand at room temperature for a couple of days, it didn't spoil. Quite to the contrary—it improved! The interaction of certain bacilli in raw milk with airborne bacteria initiated a fermentation process that soured the milk into a semi-solid pudding with a delicious sweet-sour taste and considerable nutritional benefits.

Today's pasteurized, homogenized milk, however, rots and becomes inedible if left unrefrigerated. Fresh milk and cream must always be stored in the fridge in tightly closed containers that protect milk from light, which would otherwise destroy riboflavin (vitamin B2) and vitamin B6. Unopened, milk stays fresh for two to three weeks. Keep all containers tightly closed, so the milk doesn't absorb odors from other foods. Once containers are opened, air and bacteria are introduced, making the milk more perishable. Milk from an open container, therefore, must be used within several days.

For refrigerated cultured milks, such as buttermilk, sour cream, and yogurt, stay-fresh times vary: two to three weeks for buttermilk, three to four weeks for sour cream. Yogurt maintains a fresh taste and appearance for up to six weeks. However, the number of beneficial lactic acid bacteria (LAB) in yogurt remains stable for only two to three weeks from the date of manufacture, after which it gradually declines. If you buy commercial yogurt, you can determine the approximate date of manufacture by counting back forty–five days from the "best before" date on the package.

Natural cheese is a living food. In soft cheese, especially, there are millions of microorganisms at work, but even in hard cheese, internal biochemical reactions continue as it matures and ages. All cheese must be refrigerated and is best kept in its original package, or tightly wrapped in aluminum foil or waxed paper, then placed inside a plastic bag so it has room to breathe. For cheese that has been cut, an additional layer of plastic wrap will keep it from drying out. Hard cheese that has not been cut or grated will stay fresh for up to six months. Soft cheeses (cream cheese, cottage, ricotta) should be used within a week after opening. For optimal flavor, bring cheese to room temperature before serving.

Fowl—the meat of choice

Rather than heavier types of meat, the Cayce readings recommend fowl, as this is more readily assimilated by the body:

> We would be mindful of the diet, that those foods are taken that are easily assimilated. Do not take quantities of grease of any nature . . . When meats *are* taken, they should be those either of roast beef or roast mutton, or fish, or fowl— but not fried fowl, even. It should be either baked or broiled . . .
>
> . . . Do not eat meat more than three times each week, and don't gorge self when this is done!   481-1

The readings also suggest that chewing the bony portions of fowl meats provides the body with an excellent source of easily assimilable calcium:

> . . . the lean or bony portions would be very well to supply more calcium . . . and those bony portions of [fish and fowl] that are cooked to such an extent that these may be masticated also.   1973-1

And:

> **When fowl is taken choose rather the very small bony pieces rather than what might appear to be the more delicate. Take those that are not supposed to be choice pieces—as the wimblebit, the back, the neck, the feet. All of these are much preferable and have much more vital energies for body building.** 2084-15

The parts of fowl mentioned in this reading are also excellent as a base for cooking nutrient-rich soups, broths, and stews.

One of the best fowl meats we can choose, with respect to both our health and the environment, is turkey. In contrast to chickens, cattle, or pigs, which are often forced to live in torturous, cramped conditions directly above their own excrement, turkeys are seldom reared in confinement, but are allowed to roam freely in fields and meadows.

If you have a taste for game bird, wild turkey is an excellent choice, although it tends to be more expensive. Several of the Cayce readings recommend wild game. Reading 749-1 says, "Wild game would be most preferable for the meats." Wild turkeys distinguish themselves from domestic turkeys by their high-keeled breast bones and long legs. In contrast to domestic turkeys, wild turkeys can actually fly.

Wild turkey contains less than half of the fat and cholesterol of domestic turkey. Along with wild pheasant and gray partridge, wild turkey has a protein content that is higher than that found in any other type of meat.

The meat departments in many natural food stores around the country often source organic turkeys and other wild game from local area farmers. As we have seen, local foods are best for your health and the environment, as they ensure optimal freshness and the least environmental impact in terms of packaging and transportation. If local organic turkey is not available in your area, your natural foods retailer may be able to source frozen organic wild and domestic turkeys from wholesale outlets that ship the birds frozen in temperature-controlled transport trucks.

Dangers of processed meats

If you eat any other type of meat, choose your source carefully. Most commercial meat comes from animals raised in crowded, unhealthy conditions and fed grains laced with pesticides, as well as genetically engineered soy feed. The animals have often been given growth stimulants, steroids, and antibiotics, the residues of which remain lodged in the meat. Organic meat from grass–fed animals raised in a natural environment is a much healthier choice.

Avoid cured meats, such as ham, hot dogs, sausage, bacon, and various cold cuts. These are processed meats that have been preserved with nitrites, nitrates, and other chemicals, which have been linked to cancer of the digestive tract, bladder, and lungs. In children, the frequent consumption of hot dogs and other cured meats raises the risk of brain cancer and childhood leukemia, according to research conducted at the University of North Carolina at Chapel Hill and the University of Southern California School of Medicine in Los Angeles.

Research published in the March 2002 issue of *Diabetes Care* showed that eating a diet high in processed meats may substantially increase the risk of developing type II diabetes in men. In the study, men who ate processed meats five or more times per week had a 50 percent higher risk of developing the disease.

Fish failings

Eating fish is highly recommended in the Cayce readings, especially for those suffering from glandular disturbances and obesity. Reading 3076–1 says, "In the matter of the diet for the body—keep plenty of seafoods of all characters about three times a week." This reading was given in 1943. In the twenty–first century, however, due to widespread environmental pollution, many fish contain high levels of mercury, a known neurotoxin, and other toxic pollutants. It is impossible today to recommend eating fish and other seafood without this caveat.

Consumers, therefore, are faced with a difficult choice: On the one hand, we are told that eating fish at least two or three times a week protects against heart disease, while on the other hand, we are warned against eating certain types of fish more than once a month because of their high mercury levels. Children, pregnant women, and women of childbearing age are urged to be especially cautious. High mercury levels can cause brain damage in unborn children. Farmed salmon has even been found to contain flame retardants.

The concern about fish safety should seriously alarm all of us, as it is a sad indication of how contaminated we have allowed our environment to become. We can no longer safely eat one of the healthiest, most nutritious foods offered to us by Mother Nature because we have let our oceans become harbors of toxic waste water that threatens the very existence of the creatures living in it and those higher up in the food chain—humans and land animals.

In the fall of 2006, scientists advised us that, despite high levels of toxicity, the health benefits of eating fish far outweighed the risk. But shortly after this announcement was issued, a group of researchers warned that pollution and over-fishing were wiping out the fish stocks of the world's oceans and that if we continued our current practices, all wild seafood would be gone by 2048. Even now, seafood species such as soft-shell crab, which used to be plentiful, have become rare, and this phenomenon will only increase if we don't stop polluting the oceans and cease the practices of heavy fishing that deplete one species after another.

We must change our ways. We must treat the earth and all its creatures with respect and stop looking for short-term gain while ignoring the serious damage we are doing to our planet's ecosystems. In the meantime, we need to exercise caution with respect to the types of fish we eat and how they are sourced. If we took care in this book to list the types of fish that are currently considered safe to eat, the information might no longer be up to date by the time you read it. It is best, therefore, to suggest downloading *The Green Guide*'s regularly updated Fish Picks card from the Internet: http://www.thegreenguide. com/gg/pdf/fishchartissue97.pdf. You can also visit the EPA's Fish Advisories Web page at http://www.epa.gov/waterscience/fish/ for more information on fish and fish safety.

After purchasing fish, meat, or poultry, refrigerate it immediately and keep it well-wrapped to prevent other foods from coming into contact with it. Fresh ground beef and lamb should be used within two days; other cuts may be kept refrigerated for up to five days. A greenish pigment on meat indicates spoilage due to bacterial action. Poultry and fish may be kept in the fridge for up to two days. If their odor is unpleasant or "fishy," in the case of fish, discard the product or return it to the store.

Be soy sensible

Soybeans, which are higher in protein than other plant foods, have become a popular substitute for animal protein. Some nutrition researchers, however, are concerned that not all soy products are health promoting. Soybeans are high in phytates, which inhibit the absorption of essential minerals such as calcium, magnesium, iron, and zinc. The phytate content in traditionally fermented soy products, such as tempeh or miso, is reduced; but in the more popular tofu, made from soybean curd, phytates remain high. Research has shown that vegetarian diets high in soy tend to promote iron deficiency, particularly in women.

There are few references to soy in the Cayce readings. In one case, a questioner who asked what was the best meat substitute was told, "soy beans." (257–252) In general, however, soy products in the readings are recommended with a caveat. They are said to be beneficial only for physically active individuals. When asked whether soy milk was advisable, Cayce replied: "This will depend much upon the activities of the body. If there is sufficient of the energies used for physical activities to make same more easily assimilated, it is well. If these energies are used for activities which are more mental than physical, it would not be so well." (1158–18)

Among nutrition experts, there are also concerns about soy's high content of phytoestrogens, which are plant substances that mimic hormone action in the body. In children raised on soy formula, experts have linked the increased occurrence of premature thelarche (the beginning of breast development at the onset of puberty) with soy's high phytoestrogen content. In Puerto Rico, pediatric endocrinologists found a positive association between premature sexual development and the consumption of soy formula. Girls as young as eight years of age showed breast development and pubic hair growth. Premature sexual development has been linked with an increased risk of ovarian cysts and thus ovarian cancer, and a greater lifetime risk of breast cancer.

The endocrine–disruptive action of soy phytoestrogens can also cause thyroid dysfunction in humans. As we have already seen, the thyroid is a master gland that controls endocrine activity, including the way in which the body burns fat. It is important for all who want to lose weight to ensure optimal thyroid function. It is wise, therefore, not to rely heavily on soy in the diet.

In summary, remember that protein is your friend, and as with human friendships, it's quality that counts more than quantity. We do need to eat sufficient protein to sustain the body and maintain optimal metabolic function, but we don't need nearly as much protein as many of us have come to expect on our dinner plate every day.

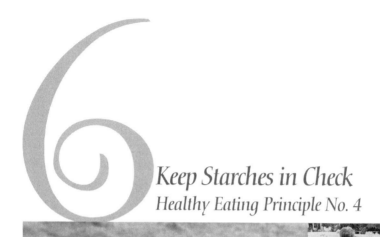

Keep Starches in Check
Healthy Eating Principle No. 4

A FOOD THAT NOT ONLY TASTES GREAT but also helps improve bowel regularity, shed extra pounds, lower cholesterol levels, and reduce the risk of diabetes—does that sound too good to be true? That food group is whole grains, and you can easily incorporate it into your diet. Breads, crackers, and cereals made with whole grains enjoy increased popularity as consumers are discovering the scrumptious flavor and nutritional value of unrefined grains. Food producers and retailers have responded by offering new food products based on whole grains. Brown rice and whole-grain pasta are showing up on menus in restaurants, delis, and cafeterias.

The Cayce readings also recommend that whole grains be included in the diet. Reading 2261-1 suggests, "Those of bread—keep those that are of the whole wheat, or those of the rye, or those of the nature that are easily assimilated, and we will find in two to three months a normal body, with the proper weight, proper adjustments, and feeling better . . ."

There is a world of difference between whole grains, which are unrefined starches, and refined starches such as white-flour products and white rice. To be sure, any type of dietary starch must be kept within limits, especially for those wanting to lose weight, but whole grains in small amounts do have a place in the healthy diet. Let's take a close look at the difference between whole grains and refined starchy foods.

What's in a grain kernel?

Whole grains provide superior nutrition because they contain the full spectrum of nutrients found in the grain kernel. A grain kernel consists of three parts: the innermost germ; the endosperm, which surrounds the germ; and the bran, which envelops both. In the refining process, the germ and bran are stripped away, leaving only the starchy endosperm, which is then ground into flour. Most of the grain kernel's nutrients, however, are locked into the germ and bran, including minerals such as magnesium and zinc, the all-important vitamin B complex, and vitamin E. B vitamins help the body break down carbohydrates, produce energy, and maintain a healthy nervous system. Vitamin E is an antioxidant that has been shown to have heart-protective and rejuvenating properties. Many people are chronically deficient in vitamin E. Eating whole grains daily is an excellent way to ensure a regular intake of this important nutrient.

Another vital constituent of whole grains is fiber, an indigestible carbohydrate that increases bulk and softness of stools, thus improving bowel regularity. Fiber acts as a natural cleanser that helps remove encrusted fecal matter and toxic debris as it travels along the intestinal pathways. Fiber also assists in controlling blood sugar levels by slowing down the rate of food passage through the intestinal tract, resulting in a more gradual release of glucose into the bloodstream. A number of recent studies, including research published in the February 2004 issue of *Diabetes Care*, have shown that a diet rich in whole grains may lower the risk of type II diabetes. Study subjects who consumed three or more servings of whole grains per day had improved insulin sensitivity, meaning that their body became more efficient at responding to insulin—a mechanism impaired in those with type II diabetes. Other research has shown fiber to be effective in reducing undesirable LDL blood cholesterol.

Optimal fiber intake ranges from thirty to forty grams per day, but the typical Western diet provides only half that amount: between ten and twenty grams per day. In our ongoing love affair with refined and packaged foods, which have been stripped of fiber, we have sacrificed one of our greatest allies in our quest for health.

Although fiber has no vitamins or minerals, it does make a nutritional contribution to the diet: Fiber serves as a food for bowel flora—the friendly bacteria that naturally reside in the intestinal tract—encouraging it to flourish and produce anti–infectious and anticarcinogenic substances. By helping keep the intestinal tract clean and the bowel flora healthy, dietary fiber also supports a strong immune system.

There are two types of fiber, each performing a specific function in the body. *Soluble fiber,* which includes pectins and gums, dissolves in fluids and forms a gel–like substance in the intestinal tract, thus helping soften stools and facilitating their expulsion. Soluble fiber helps reduce serum cholesterol levels by binding intestinal bile acids that contain fat and cholesterol, ensuring that these are removed in the stools instead of being reabsorbed into the bloodstream. This beneficial effect may help reduce the risk of cardiovascular disease.

Insoluble fiber, which includes cellulose, hemicellulose, and lignins, soaks up water like a sponge and acts as a bulking agent, speeding up the time it takes for fecal waste to be moved through the intestinal tract. This helps prevent constipation, as well as more serious bowel conditions such as diverticulosis, in which small pouches form in the large intestine, trapping fecal matter. Most unrefined plant foods contain a balance of soluble and insoluble fiber, which act together to provide optimal gelling and bulking in the intestinal tract.

The glycemic index

The glycemic index ranks carbohydrates based on their immediate effect on blood sugar levels. Carbohydrates that break down quickly during digestion have the highest values, whereas carbohydrates that break down slowly and release sugars gradually into the bloodstream have the lowest values. Refined sugars and starches appear high on the glycemic index, whereas most vegetables and whole grains occupy a much lower ranking.

A study published in the November 24, 2004, issue of the *Journal of the American Medical Association* demonstrated that a diet that emphasizes foods ranking low on the glycemic index promotes greater weight loss than a diet based on high–glycemic foods. A study in the February 15, 2005, *American Journal of Epidemiology* confirmed that the type of carbohydrates we consume determines whether we are prone to gaining weight or keeping it off. The study found that overweight people tend to eat more refined carbs, such as white bread and pasta. An earlier study conducted in 2004 by a team of researchers at cereal–maker General Mills had also found that individuals who ate three or more daily servings of whole grains were the least likely to be overweight or obese. The company subsequently decided to begin using whole grains in all of its breakfast cereals.

Although the glycemic index had not yet been invented when Cayce suggested that an excess of starchy and refined foods in the diet was a major contributor to obesity, the readings' advice is largely aligned with what researchers have determined about high– and low–glycemic foods. We must realize that we cannot continue to eat refined foods and expect to keep healthy and slim. Natural whole foods contain all the vitamins, minerals, and phytochemicals required to nourish the body and promote good health, but only a small fraction of these remain in refined foods. In our efforts to achieve a more natural weight for our bodies, we are wise to base our diet on whole, unrefined, and unprocessed foods.

For optimal digestibility and assimilation of whole grains, they should be thoroughly soaked before cooking. Whole grains are high in phytic acid, which blocks the absorption of minerals. They also contain enzyme inhibitors, which protect the plant from sprouting prematurely. These enzyme inhibitors, however, make unsprouted grains difficult to digest. Soaking or sour–leavening helps neutralize the phytic acid and enzyme inhibitors. Bread made with sourdough, therefore, is easier to digest.

Label of truth. When shopping for whole–grain products, remember that products labeled "multi-grain," "stone–ground," or "bran" are not automatically whole–grain products and that a darker color does not necessarily indicate an unrefined product. Bread, for instance, might appear brown because of added molasses. Be sure the label says "100% whole grain," or at least that a whole–grain ingredient such as "whole wheat," "whole rye," or "whole oats" is listed as the first item on the label.

Alternative Grains

With the increasing incidence of wheat allergies, many people are looking for healthy alternatives that can be used in much the same way as wheat. The ancient, nonhybridized relatives of our modern staple grains are flavorful, richly textured, and highly nutritious. Look for the following popular alternative grains in your health food store.

Amaranth. A sacred food of the ancient Aztecs, amaranth has a distinctive nutty taste. The tiny, light–colored grains can be cooked as breakfast cereal or added to other cereals and soups for extra flavor and thickness. Use amaranth flour as you would regular wheat flour. It is nonglutinous and safe for those with gluten sensitivities. Amaranth is high in protein, fiber, B vitamins, and minerals, including calcium, magnesium, zinc, copper, and iron.

Kamut. The rich, buttery flavor of this ancient Egyptian grain and relative of durum wheat makes kamut a popular substitute for regular wheat. Cook kamut whole, as you would the wheat berry, for cereal. Kamut flour is great for baking breads and healthful snacks, and for making pasta. Kamut contains all eight essential amino acids, which makes it a complete protein. It is also high in fiber, vitamins B and E, and several minerals.

Millet. Popular in Asian and African cuisine, millet has a mild, nutty flavor and creamy texture. It is very satisfying as a cooked breakfast cereal on a cold winter morning. Millet is a unique grain because it helps alkalize the body, whereas most other grains are acid–forming when metabolized. Millet provides protein, fiber, B vitamins, and iron, as well as lecithin and choline, which help maintain a healthy cholesterol profile.

Quinoa. The ancient Incas called quinoa the "mother grain" and considered it a sacred food. Quinoa has been cultivated in the rugged highlands of South America for centuries. Use mild–flavored quinoa as you would rice—as a side dish or in salads, such as tabbouleh or vegetable pilaf. Rinse grains well before cooking to remove their natural resin coating. Quinoa offers complete protein, fiber, B vitamins, and minerals, including magnesium, potassium, manganese, and zinc.

Spelt. This ancient grain dates back to biblical times, as it is mentioned by name in Exodus, Isaiah, and Ezekiel. Saint Hildegard of Bingen, a twelfth-century mystic, recommended it for those too weak to eat other foods. Spelt is a rich source of easily assimilable nutrients, including protein and lignins. It also contains immune stimulants and anticarcinogenic phytochemicals. Sweet-tasting spelt and spelt flour can be substituted in recipes calling for wheat or rice.

Wild rice. A staple food of native Canadians, wild rice has an aromatic, woodsy flavor. It is higher in protein, minerals, and B vitamins than common rice. It can be substituted for rice in recipes or added to regular rice to spice up its flavor and texture.

These wholesome and tasty wheat alternatives will introduce you to a whole new way of experiencing your meals and will effectively support your health and your weight-loss goals!

Think whole salt

The modern food industry has changed the way we think of food. When we say "salt," for instance, we typically visualize tiny, white, free-flowing crystals, and when we say "sugar," a similar picture comes to mind. But this type of even texture and flawless white color is the result of several steps of processing and refining. It's not how salt and sugar occur in nature.

Common table salt is made from refined rock salt that has been stripped of its natural mineral balance, reducing it to 99 percent sodium chloride. The rest is additives—bleaching and free-flowing agents, stabilizers, and aluminum compounds. Even sea salt, if it's white and free-flowing, has been highly refined, removing essential minerals and trace elements. Like common table salt, refined sea salt is mostly sodium chloride and contains no other nutrients.

Whole, unrefined sea salt, available in health food stores, is light gray in color. Because it is hand-harvested and naturally dried by the sun and air rather than through the artificial heat of a kiln, it retains a moist, lumpy texture. Unprocessed sea salt contains more than eighty essential minerals and trace elements that closely resemble the constituents of human body fluids—blood, lymph, sweat, and tears are all salty.

The essential trace mineral iodine is present in unrefined sea salt in a form that is easily assimilated. Iodine is a vital constituent of the hormones produced by the thyroid gland, which controls several biochemical reactions, including oxygen utilization, protein synthesis, and the rate at which the body burns food. The refining process destroys the iodine in white sea salt. An inorganic form of iodine, most often potassium iodide, is added to refined table salt. However, this type of iodine is not readily assimilated by the body. It passes in the urine quickly, usually within twenty minutes, whereas natural iodine from unrefined sea salt is retained for forty-eight hours—long enough to be utilized by the thyroid. Unrefined sea salt can even help normalize blood pressure by breaking down fats and cholesterol in the arteries and promoting good circulation.

Naturally sweet and wholesome

Like refined salt, white sugar has been stripped of all the vitamins, minerals, and trace elements that naturally occur in the whole sugar cane plant. The whole plant contains only 14 percent sucrose, along with fiber, water, and various other nutrients. The refining process separates the sugar from the molasses, the nutrient-rich part of the sugar plant. Refined, white sugar is pure sucrose. Brown sugar is refined sugar that has some of the molasses added back to it, mostly for color. It is still a refined sugar product.

Health food stores offer a wide selection of natural sweeteners that are excellent whole-food alternatives to refined cane sugar. Enjoyed in moderation, they form a wholesome part of a healthy diet:

- **Sucanat** is dehydrated sugar cane juice which contains the nutrient-rich molasses that refining typically removes. Sucanat is high in chromium, which helps balance blood sugar, and also provides many other important minerals, including magnesium, silica, and iron. It can be substituted for sugar in any recipe.
- **Date sugar** is made from whole, pulverized dates. It is highly

nutritious and provides vitamins, minerals, and fiber. Truly a whole food, date sugar comes with a high price tag, but offers a fabulous nutrient profile in return.

- **Raw honey**, available in health food stores, has a long history of use as a medicinal food for various ailments, including colds, coughs, and digestive difficulties. Along with its naturally sweet taste, honey offers small amounts of protein, vitamins, minerals, and enzymes. Never buy pasteurized honey, whose enzymes have been destroyed by heat. Make sure your honey is from a reputable source and does not come from sugar–fed bees.

Maple syrup, barley malt, stevia, and rice syrup are other whole–food alternatives that can be used in place of refined sugar.

The Cayce readings explain that it is the combination of sugars and starches, rather than the sugars themselves, that are acid–producing and thus harmful. A 47–year–old man who asked about starches and sweets, received the following answer:

> **As has been indicated, these are not to be entirely tabu, but as would be from a normal mental balance of consideration, take about eighty percent alkalin-producing foods to twenty percent acid-producing. Sugars are in *main*, combined with starches, acid-producing. Starches also produce energy, as does sugar. It is the combinations of these that become rather as hindrances, than the *individual* properties themselves, see?** 877-28

A 57–year–old woman with a tendency toward obesity was told:

> **Do not combine *any* of starches with any quantities of sweets. Do not take food values that cause great quantity of alcoholic reaction. This does not refer to alcohol, but sweets and certain starches produce a character of fermentation that is alcoholic that makes for excess of fatty portions for the body.** 1125-2

The Cayce readings consider beet sugar to be the best type of sugar, with raw honey or unrefined cane sugar the best substitutes. Beet sugar[3] is often difficult to find, and Sucanat, the unrefined whole sugar listed above, is an excellent alternative.

Remember that excess sugars being converted into body fat is how weight gain occurs in the first place. Therefore, anyone looking to lose weight would do well to limit sugars and especially refined starches, which rapidly convert to sugar in the body.

Breakfast: an epiphany

Many people who are trying to lose weight believe that skipping breakfast is one of the ways in which they can reach their goal more quickly. Skipping the morning meal, they feel, helps them cut out calories from their overall daily intake. Yet numerous studies have shown that breakfast is important for optimal physical and mental performance. Eating a nutritious meal in the morning also boosts metabolism, which determines the rate at which the body burns food. Breakfast also promotes mental alertness and emotional stability throughout the day.

A study reported in the November 2001 issue of the *American Journal of Clinical Nutrition* showed that eating breakfast improved memory performance in elderly test subjects. A year earlier, research conducted by Harvard University had demonstrated that schools that offer free breakfast to their students reported higher math scores and lower absenteeism. Students participating in breakfast programs were better-behaved and registered improved math scores.

These and similar studies have made it clear that people of every age can benefit from eating a good breakfast. Whether you spend your day in an office, in a school, at home, or in an outdoor environment, your morning will be more productive if you start the day with a nourishing meal. If you skip breakfast, you'll experience hunger pangs throughout the morning, which may cause you to snack more frequently in order to shake this uncomfortable feeling. Breakfast skippers tend to consume low-nutrient snack foods more frequently during the day. One reason is that the appetite is partly regulated by blood sugar levels. Without

---

[3] Beet sugar is available from Baar Products Inc., baar.com.

breakfast, blood sugar levels don't become sufficiently elevated in the morning, prompting the body to produce constant "hunger" signals. This, in turn, causes us to eat more than we actually need.

The same reaction occurs when a typical weekday breakfast of fruit juice and coffee with toast and jam is eaten! High in sugar, starch, and caffeine, this meal provides just enough quick energy to help fight one's way through rush–hour traffic. By the time many folks get to work, their blood sugar levels have dropped and they feel edgy or tired and need another caffeine fix, this time taken with a donut!

To ensure optimal energy and mental alertness throughout the day, always eat a nourishing breakfast emphasizing whole foods that are metabolized slowly, so that you won't experience major blood sugar fluctuations.

The Cayce readings recommend a variety of wholesome breakfast foods, including coddled egg with lightly buttered whole–wheat toast, and well–cooked whole–grain cereals, such as steel–cut oats. Citrus fruits and their juices are also suggested for the morning meal, but are never to be combined with cereals except a single slice of whole–wheat toast. Otherwise, combining citrus fruits or juices with cereals is said to create unfavorable acidic conditions in the body.

The readings consider the moderate consumption of coffee or tea to be acceptable for most people, although coffee is said to have a higher food value. The addition of milk or cream to either coffee or tea is not recommended, since this increases the acidity. During the past several years, many studies involving coffee have been published. The results are extremely variable, suggesting on the one hand that coffee could help prevent serious conditions such as Parkinson's disease, liver damage, and diabetes, while on the other hand, it could promote heart problems. On average, however, most of these studies seem to agree with Cayce that, taken in moderation, coffee is not harmful and may even have a wide range of benefits. If you drink coffee, be sure to take it with or after food. Taken on an empty stomach, the caffeine in coffee could wreak havoc with your nervous system!

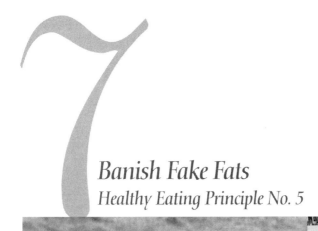

Banish Fake Fats

Healthy Eating Principle No. 5

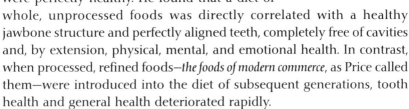

THE LATE WESTON A. PRICE, a dentist and nutrition pioneer, traveled the world in search of people and ethnic groups who were perfectly healthy. He found that a diet of whole, unprocessed foods was directly correlated with a healthy jawbone structure and perfectly aligned teeth, completely free of cavities and, by extension, physical, mental, and emotional health. In contrast, when processed, refined foods—*the foods of modern commerce*, as Price called them—were introduced into the diet of subsequent generations, tooth health and general health deteriorated rapidly.

Price documented his findings in the book *Nutrition and Physical Degeneration.* Specifically, he established that ethnic cultures who were highly particular about their organic farming practices and whose dairy farmers, for instance, made it a priority to increase the fat content of cows' milk, enjoyed better health than ethnic groups who were not as meticulous in their farming techniques. This led Price to conclude that humans achieve perfect physical form and perfect health, generation after generation, only when they consume nutrient-dense whole foods and the vital fat–soluble activators found exclusively in animal fats.

These fat–soluble activators are essential for the assimilation of vitamins A, D, and E, and vital minerals such as calcium. Whole milk, as we have seen in chapter five, includes the proper balance of fats to ensure optimal utilization of these nutrients. Fermented whole milks, such as yogurt and kefir, are the most bioavailable. The body is unable to fully utilize the calcium and other nutrients from low–fat and skim milks.

Cod liver oil and butter from pasture–fed cows were highly regarded by Price for their value in delivering easily assimilable vitamins A and D to the body and in optimizing immune function.

One of Price's associates, Francis Pottenger, observed in research involving cats that when one generation began eating *the foods of modern commerce*, especially refined carbohydrates (white sugar, white flour, white rice), their offspring (generation 1) began to have crowded, crooked, bad teeth. The subsequent generation (2) suffered from allergies, followed by autoimmune diseases in generation 3. The following generation (4) displayed sociological problems, mental illness, endocrine problems, and infertility.

Modern physicians who have worked with Price's research have found that inadequate calcium intake and assimilation as a result of processed foods and reduced intake of whole fats have caused an average 30–percent reduction in bone density in modern humans. This, in turn, has led to inadequate jawbone and tooth structure formation, as well as tooth decay. Perfectly healthy teeth are rarely seen in the industrialized world. The teeth of many of today's children are growing in unevenly, appearing crooked or protruding horizontally on either side of the gums, instead of straight and vertically. This is the same phenomenon that was observed in generation 1 of Pottenger's cat experiment.

Allergies and autoimmune diseases are ubiquitous today and increasing at alarming rates. The incidence of infertility in American couples at age twenty–five currently stands at 30 percent—symptoms that are equivalent to those observed in generation 4 of Pottenger's cats. It appears that this is nature's way of telling us we've gone too far and can't allow the situation to continue.

Our widespread, inappropriate fear of healthy fats is one of the factors that has contributed to this unhealthy situation. Producers of margarine and commercial vegetable oils have persuaded many consumers to give up natural fats such as butter, which has a long history of safe use. Instead, we are told to choose manufactured fats that are refined, bleached, deodorized, and loaded with substances far worse than the natural fats they are intended to replace.

Remember that eating a whole-foods diet does not mean depriving yourself of fats. It means choosing the right fats in moderation—natural, unrefined fats, which are a concentrated source of energy and play an important role in metabolism and in protecting cellular health. The fat-soluble vitamins A, D, E, and K and the carotenoids depend on the presence of dietary fats for their assimilation. Such natural fats are also precursors of hormones and hormone-like chemicals called prostaglandins.

Butter is better

Butter, especially butter from pasture-fed cows, is an excellent source of natural fats and fat-soluble vitamins, notably vitamin A, which helps support optimal immune function and the health of the endocrine system. Lecithin, a natural emulsifying agent found in butter, ensures the proper assimilation of cholesterol.

Butter has been safely used as a staple food and versatile culinary fat throughout history. Remember that butter is not meat fat. It contains not only saturated fats but also healthy monounsaturated fatty acids and traces of the essential fatty acids that our bodies need. And as far as saturated fats are concerned, expert opinions diverge on their effects on the body. Many progressive nutritionists refute the assumption that natural saturated fats, which have a long tradition of dietary use, cause cardiovascular disease, referring instead to the correlation between the increase of refined vegetable oils and other processed foods in the diet and the corresponding increase in heart disease.

Butter has been unjustly implicated in promoting disease that should be blamed on processed foods. It has been villainized by market-share-hungry producers of margarine and vegetable shortening, both of which are unhealthy, manufactured fats. Unfortunately, many medical doctors, who for the most part have little or no training in nutrition, have believed the manufacturers' claims and unwittingly helped promote their unhealthful products.

The Cayce readings recommend butter in moderation, as a seasoning on vegetables or as a spread on toast. Reading 3033-1 says: "Of course, butter may be taken. And the vegetables should be prepared preferably with butter if any seasoning is to be used . . ." In another reading, a 53-year-old woman who complained about nerve pain below her shoulder blades was told that she needed to include more butterfats or dairy fats in her diet.

Butter is easily digested and does not put any strain on the liver. This makes it a good fat for anyone, including those with digestive problems.

Olive oil—queen among oils

Olive oil has long been valued by gourmet chefs, food lovers, and nutritionists alike. Tasty, versatile, and rich in health-giving nutrients, it is a culinary oil par excellence. Olive oil makes a delicious base for salad dressings, dips, and sauces. Because its fatty acids are mostly monounsaturated, olive oil is stable when heated and is therefore safe for use in cooking and baking.

For best quality and flavor, be sure to choose *extra virgin olive oil*, which is produced from the first pressing of olives, using a mechanical process that does not employ heat or solvents. Oil from the second pressing is known as *virgin olive oil*. The next grade down is *pure olive oil*, which is produced through heat extraction. Still lower grades, extracted with chemical solvents, are labeled "olive oil" and "light" or "lite olive oil." These are refined olive oils that have lost much of the goodness of the natural product. They are also more acidic. Read labels carefully and avoid these refined olive oils and all other solvent-processed oils.

Olive oil plays an important role in the Mediterranean diet, which has been credited with helping people live longer, healthier lives. Many studies have been done in hopes of identifying the specific components of the diet that are responsible for its health benefits. Recent research has focused on the anti-inflammatory effects of extra-virgin olive oil that were found to be equivalent to those of the well-known anti-inflammatory drug ibuprofen.

Earlier studies had shown that olive oil helps keep the heart young and prevent circulatory diseases and high blood pressure. Some of olive oil's benefits may be due to its high content of vitamin E and flavonoid-rich phenols, which offer powerful antioxidant action.

Olive oil also stimulates bile secretion and strengthens liver function. In combination with lemon juice, it is often used in liver cleanses and in the prevention and treatment of gallstones.

The Cayce readings recommend olive oil for culinary use as well as for medicinal purposes. Taken in small quantities throughout the day—several drops to a half teaspoonful every few hours—it is said to be soothing for the entire intestinal tract. Reading 3842-1 says: "We would take all the olive oil we are able to assimilate, in very small doses. This may be taken two, three, four, five times each day—half a teaspoonful . . ." And reading 846-1 advises: "Olive oil in *small* quantities is *always* good for the whole of the intestinal system."

An article in the November 2003 issue of *Meridian Institute News* (www.meridianinstitute.com) titled "Can olive oil help acid reflux?" tells the story of someone who used the Cayce–recommended small doses of extra–virgin olive oil to successfully treat symptoms of acid reflux that occurred following surgery for gallbladder removal. Longtime A.R.E. volunteer Nancy Thomas followed the recommendations of the article and was equally successful in curing her acid reflux and related symptoms. She shared her success story about this and other Cayce therapies in an article she wrote for the Spring 2007 issue of *Spa Life* magazine (www.spalifemagazine.com).

In October 2006, a group of physicians from Attikon University Hospital in Athens, Greece, in a letter to the *European Journal of Gastro-enterology and Hepatology*, reported on seven patients who had undergone a gastrectomy (the removal of all or part of the stomach) and subsequently used a treatment consisting of a spoonful of olive oil several times a day for the severe reflux symptoms that typically follow gastrectomy. All of the patients improved; three no longer experienced any reflux symptoms, while four showed a significant improvement.

In 2007, researchers from the Spanish Institute de la Grasa, and the University Hospital of Valme, demonstrated that polyphenols found in olive oil may prevent infection with the *Helicobacter pylori* bacteria, which is believed to be a major cause of gastritis and peptic ulcers. Reported in the *Journal of Agricultural and Food Chemistry* (Vol. 55, pp. 680–6), the study considers extra–virgin olive oil to be a potential chemoprotective agent for peptic ulcer and gastric cancer.

Extra–virgin olive oil is truly a wonder food and a versatile home remedy that should be a staple in every natural foods kitchen! If you've run out, however, there are some alternatives. Avocado oil, macadamia nut oil, coconut oil, and almond oil are other stable culinary oils that do not easily spoil and turn rancid. They may be used in place of olive oil or butter in cooking and baking. Coconut oil and almond oil have a mildly sweet flavor that combines well with baked goods.

Beware of fake oils

Avoid the clean–looking, refined, processed vegetable oils found on supermarket shelves. Most often, these oils have been extracted with the use of heat and solvents, and have been bleached and deodorized to improve the oils' appearance and to neutralize odor and taste. These oils are chemically unstable—they are polyunsaturated, which makes them vulnerable to molecular damage and rancidity.

Further damage is done when vegetable oils are artificially hardened by hydrogenation. Hydrogenated fats are found in margarines, vegetable oil shortenings, commercial baked goods, and processed foods and snacks. These are true junk foods because they contain trans–fatty acids, which are chemically altered molecules that disrupt the function of enzymes and metabolic processes in the body.

Research has established beyond a doubt that trans–fatty acids are damaging to our health and contribute to cardiovascular problems and degenerative disease. The food industry today has come under pressure to reduce and eliminate trans–fatty acids in their products, but it will likely be a long haul until these goals are accomplished, particularly because the common misconception about natural fats such as butter prevails. So, the onus remains on us to read labels carefully and to make sure we avoid dangerous manufactured fats and trans–fatty acids.

Fats that boost metabolism

If you are trying to lose weight, you may be tempted to avoid all dietary fats, but this is not a helpful step because it could seriously disrupt metabolic function and ultimately sabotage your weight-loss efforts. The fats you eat are not automatically converted to body fat—in fact, certain fats help burn it off. The omega-3 fatty acids, often missing from the modern diet but abundantly present in flax seeds, are particularly effective at correcting the body's thermogenic processes. Add freshly ground flax seeds to cereals or soups, or take cold-pressed, unrefined flax seed oil (1–3 tablespoons daily). Flax seed oil is also good to use in salad dressings. Be sure to refrigerate any unused portions immediately, and never heat the oil or use it in cooking, as it is extremely heat sensitive.

Unrefined coconut oil is a rich source of medium-chain triglycerides, which burn up quickly in the body. They increase metabolic rate and thus promote weight loss. Tasty coconut oil adds delicious exotic flavor to many dishes and baked goods. It also tastes great on its own. Take two to three teaspoons of coconut oil daily to help kick-start your metabolism into burning fat more readily. Unrefined pumpkin seed and walnut oils, as well as oil of evening primrose, are also high in fatty acids that help the body burn fat and calories.

Healthy and nutty

Nuts, too, are a good source of omega-3 fats and a rich source of important nutrients, providing fiber, magnesium, potassium, folic acid, and vitamin E—all of which have been shown to play an important role in preserving heart health. Eating nuts appears to be effective at keeping weight down: research has shown that those who frequently eat nuts are less often overweight than those who do not. A study out of Purdue University found that snacks of nuts, as well as seeds, help control appetite during the meal that follows, because they are satisfying and tend to reduce hunger. And, of course, as we have just seen, the omega-3 fats found in nuts help adjust the body's thermogenic mechanism.

Our most popular "nut," the peanut, is not technically a nut, but belongs in the legume family, along with dried beans and peas. Legumes contain soluble fiber, which is associated with lowered cholesterol and triglycerides, and decreased risk of heart attacks. The peanut is highly nutritious, providing protein, B vitamins, vitamin E, iron, calcium, and potassium. Choose organic peanuts whenever possible, as conventional varieties often have high levels of pesticide residues.

Research suggests that walnuts and almonds have a beneficial effect on blood cholesterol levels. A University of Toronto study published in the September 10, 2002, issue of *Circulation: Journal of the American Heart Association* showed that study subjects who consumed an ounce of almonds on a daily basis lowered their undesirable LDL cholesterol by 4.4 percent.

Almonds are frequently recommended in the Cayce readings for their rich nutritional profile but also for cancer prevention. Several readings suggest that eating two or three almonds each day could prevent tumor formation. Reading 1158-31, for instance, says, ". . . those who would eat two to three almonds each day need never fear cancer."

A recent study conducted at Tufts University in California showed that almonds contain very high levels of disease–fighting antioxidants, especially catechin, epicatechin, and kaempferol, which are particularly potent in fighting cell damage that can lead to illness and degenerative conditions.

A student of the Cayce readings can't help but rejoice when scientific research, in 2006, appears to substantiate what the readings said in the early part of the previous century and when once again the nutritional recommendations from the readings are proving accurate and reliable.

8

Treats to Slim Down With

IF YOU ARE LIKE MOST PEOPLE, you will sometimes find yourself with insufficient time in your day to prepare a proper meal. With increasing frequency, snacks are eaten as meal substitutes. Whether you are rushing from the office to an evening class or are chauffeuring your kids or grandchildren to one of the myriad of activities that keep us busy today, there may be occasions when you are in need of a snack that not only satisfies hunger but also your nutritional needs without causing you to pack on extra pounds.

Let's look at some yummy, nutritious snacks that we can feel good about eating, whether at home or on the run.

Fruit and veggie power

Eating sliced fruit or veggie sticks is a great way to get your daily quota of this important food group. If you're too busy to cut up your own, purchase them already prepared and ready to eat. For an even more portable and less perishable snack, choose from the wide variety of delicious dried fruit bars offered in natural food stores and some supermarkets. Fruit snacks offer concentrated vitamins and minerals, including iron. Be sure the dried fruit you purchase is organic, as sulfites and pesticide residues from nonorganic fruit are concentrated in the snack as well. Some of the organic fruit bars in health food stores are formulated with vegetables and green food concentrates for superior nutrition.

Nuts, seeds, and cereal bars

Nuts are flavorful, satisfying, and high in nutrients, including fiber, heart-healthy omega-3 fatty acids, and vitamin E, as well as magnesium, potassium, and folic acid. Some of the energy and protein bars available today are based on nuts and seeds; for instance, sesame seeds, which are a good source of calcium. The addition of whole grains, such as oats, in a cereal/nut bar, complements the protein profile of nuts and seeds. Added dried fruits, such as raisins, apricots, or dates, provide extra flavor and nutrients. Energy bars are the most popular snack food with adults, and for good reason—they pack a powerful nutritional punch!

Edgar Cayce's Mummy Food

In 1937, Edgar Cayce had a dream in which an Egyptian mummy who had come to life translated Egyptian records for him and gave him a recipe for what students of the readings today know as *Mummy Food*. The recipe called for a mixture of equal parts dates and figs to be cooked with cornmeal and water to make a smooth consistency.

Later, in a follow-up reading, guidance was sought about Cayce's dream, and once again, preparation instructions for the mixture were given exactly as in the dream. Several other readings also recommend this concoction of foods, which, according to reading 5257-1, formed "the basis of the foods of the Atlanteans and the Egyptians—corn meals with figs and dates prepared together with goat's milk."

The readings suggest that this food will have a cleansing effect on the digestive system and can help strengthen the body. Reading 2050-1 says, "Such a dish as a part of the diet often will be as an aid to better eliminations, as well as carrying those properties that will aid in building better conditions throughout the alimentary canal."

An intriguing comment proposes that the mixture "should be almost a spiritual food for the body," while another one suggests that "it's food for such a spiritually developed body as this!" (275-45)

A food that supports a person's spirituality or is especially appropriate for a spiritual person? How fascinating! What makes Mummy Food more spiritual than, say, apples and raisins?

Dates and figs are both mentioned in the Bible, although figs more frequently than dates. In 2 Kings 20:7, a poultice of figs prescribed by Isaiah heals the ailing Hezekiah. Both dates and figs are among the oldest-known domesticated foods. Dates are believed to have originated in the Persian Gulf area and appear to have been cultivated for some seven thousand years. In the spring of 2006, research published in the journal *Science* reported evidence that figs were likely to have been the first domesticated crop—as long as 11,400 years ago.

Nutritionists value both dates and figs for their impressive nutrient profile, which features abundant calcium, magnesium, potassium, and iron, as well as several vitamins. Dates tone the liver and strengthen the body. Figs are known for their gentle bulking and laxative properties, which promote cleansing and detoxification. Dried figs, in fact, contain more dietary fiber than prunes. Their calcium content even exceeds that of cows' milk. In Europe, fig syrup is a popular remedy for the relief of constipation.

The humble corn meal, too, is a good source of fiber and is helpful in the treatment of irritable bowel syndrome and other intestinal conditions. Like dates and figs, corn supplies key nutrients such as calcium, iron, magnesium, and potassium, along with other important minerals, vitamins, and phytochemicals.

It is striking that the major nutrients offered in Mummy Food are precisely those in which many people today are deficient. Calcium, magnesium, and potassium combine to strengthen muscle function and coordinate the central nervous system; they help to relax, promote restful sleep, and combat stress. Iron is important for energy production and normal brain function. All of these minerals also promote an alkaline environment in the body, which strengthens the immune system and supports all metabolic functions.

The special combination of all three foods, including the natural sugars they provide, may well increase, in ways that science cannot yet define or duplicate, these helpful qualities. Recent research confirms that it is the synergistic effect produced by all elements of a varied whole-foods diet, rather than its individual components in isolation, that results in its ability to heal and protect against illness and degenerative disease.

Mummy Food is not only healthy, it also tastes delicious. Here is the recipe, quoted from the readings:

> **1 cup Black Figs, chopped or ground very fine;**
> **1 cup Dates [remove seeds];**
> **1/2 cup Yellow Corn Meal (not too finely ground).**
>
> **Cook this for twenty minutes in sufficient water (2 or 3 cups) for it to be the consistency of mush, or cook until the meal is thoroughly cooked in same. Eat a tablespoonful of this mixture of an evening, not all at once but let it be taken slowly so as to be well assimilated as it is taken. This will be most helpful for the body.**　　　　　　　**1779-4**

Mummy food tastes especially delicious if served with milk or cream, but it is easily turned into a nutritious portable snack by placing desired amounts of the mixture into a small food container.

Easy snacks

Keep a selection of other nutritious snacks available in the fridge, at home or at work. Here are some suggestions:

- Bananas
- Fresh or dried pieces of fruit
- Medium-boiled eggs
- Whole-grain crackers
- Natural cheese
- Small tubs of yogurt or kefir

Chocolate: A new health food?

Can you slim down with chocolate? Perhaps not easily, but chocolate has gained new respect in recent years, as research has shown its main ingredient, cocoa, to be rich in antioxidant flavonoids, which help keep undesirable LDL cholesterol in check and protect the arteries. Cocoa-rich dark chocolate has higher concentrations of flavonoids than milk chocolate. Cocoa is also high in phosphorus, iron, and vitamin E, as well as other essential minerals, including potassium. Cocoa also contains a mild heart stimulant and phytochemicals that help to relax muscles and cope with stress. Occasional chocolate cravings may signal greater requirements of those nutrients.

Remember, however, that not all chocolate is created equal. Some types of chocolate are made with organically produced cocoa and other natural, wholesome ingredients, including evaporated whole sugar cane and, in the case of milk chocolate, organic milk. They are far more nutritious than many commercial chocolate varieties that are high in refined sugar and artificial flavorings, and are often produced with chemically extracted, refined vegetable oils.

Whether you use snacks to suit your busy schedule, to satisfy hunger, or just to indulge occasionally, you don't need to resort to junk food. There are many delicious, nutritious alternatives that you can safely enjoy and feel good about.

Get Physical—
The Surefire Way to Burn Fat Fast

IF YOU ARE SERIOUS ABOUT LOSING weight and getting your body into shape, you cannot escape the issue of physical activity. Several studies have shown that exercise can make a major contribution toward weight loss, including promoting the reduction of visceral fat—the fat that accumulates around the abdominal organs. Large stores of belly fat have been specifically associated with increasing the risk of diabetes and heart disease.

The results of a study published in the August 2006 issue of the *International Journal of Obesity* suggest that exercise may "preferentially increase" the body's breakdown of fat cells in the abdomen. A previous study reported in the October 2005 issue of the *Journal of Applied Physiology* produced similar results. Even moderate exercise, such as brisk walking, prevented the accumulation of further fat in the abdominal area, while those who exercised more intensely—engaging in physical activity levels equivalent to jogging twenty miles per week—shed both visceral fat and more superficial layers of abdominal fat.

Clearly, exercise is an indispensable component of any health and weight-loss program. The Cayce readings stress the importance of exercise, stating in reading 5718-1 that "the body should exercise sufficiently to at times be *physically* tired." It appears that even in Cayce's time, people were prone to overexercising the mind while underexercising the body.

In the cyber age, this tendency is not about to change, so we must make a conscious effort to include physical activity in our daily lives on a regular basis. Many of us fear that we are already too busy to devote a chunk of our precious time to exercise. If we carry additional weight on our hips or bellies, we may also feel awkward and uncomfortable at the thought of joining a fitness club and exposing our physical imperfections.

The amazing blessing is that some of the best ways to exercise are those that require neither a fitness club membership nor fancy body tights. Instead, they may require a breaking of old habits and a shift in our daily routine, such as taking the stairs instead of the elevator. This, in fact, is a new approach taken by Japan's Ministry of Health, where staff and visitors to the Ministry's twenty-six-story building in downtown Tokyo are greeted by a sign in the elevator lobby urging them to "Please use the stairs." This serves the dual purpose of providing exercise while also conserving energy, and it represents a shift in a direction that will ensure a more sustainable use of resources and energy by people everywhere.

It seems ironic that our sedentary lifestyles and our increasing reliance on cars for transportation have caused us to burn more fossil fuel while our bodies sit idle, burning less and less fuel in the form of fat and sugar and instead accumulating weight. We pay for this fossil fuel in at least two ways: first, with our hard-earned money at the gas pump, and second, with our health, not only because of our inactivity and the resulting weight gain, but also as a consequence of environmental pollution. Instead of burning more fuel driving our cars to the fitness club, we could simply leave our car in the garage or driveway and get back to basics and walk! I'm not suggesting that walking can fully meet all our transportation needs, but it can meet most of our exercise needs. There goes the excuse of not exercising because we are afraid to expose our physical imperfections at the fitness club!

Walk weight away

According to Cayce, "Walking is the best exercise!" (715-1) Several recent studies demonstrating the many health benefits of walking support Cayce's claim. With walking, limitless opportunities for getting into shape are right at your doorstep. Most of us have the option to walk, free of cost, wherever and whenever our circumstances and our schedules allow it. And other than a pair of comfortable shoes and appropriate clothing, there is no need to invest in expensive equipment or pay exorbitant club membership fees. What's more, walking usually gets us out of doors, into the open air and pumping oxygen.

Our bodies are designed to walk, and each time we do, we help increase our body's strength and vitality, as well as its ability to burn fat, even while at rest. The following are some of the benefits we can expect when we make walking part of our daily routine; here is what walking does:

- Burns calories and increases fat-burning ability
- Reduces abdominal fat
- Strengthens bones and back muscles
- Strengthens and tones leg muscles and butt
- Strengthens tendons and ligaments
- Optimizes heart and lung function
- Increases oxygen uptake
- Improves circulation
- Lowers blood pressure
- Reduces cholesterol levels
- Reduces damaging effects of stress
- Promotes healthy brain function
- Improves mood and outlook on life

Just how does walking increase the body's fat-burning ability? Muscle action draws on two types of energy—sugar and fat. Blood sugar, or glucose, is stored in the muscles; when the body moves, glucose is the first fuel to be burned, but it runs out quickly, and a steadier source of energy is required for sustained muscle activity. This is where fat comes in. Fat is stored in deposits around the visceral organs, but also in more prominently visible deposits such as the abdominal area, the hips, or the buttocks. The problem is that this fat isn't as easily accessible as glucose, especially when you've been inactive for a long time and are just beginning to work out. During long periods of inactivity, the body seems to forget how to access stored fats for energy. Although trickles of fatty acids, into which the fat molecules are broken down, are constantly released from fat cells, it isn't until we exercise for a sustained period of time that our muscles coax fat cells into letting go of larger stores of fat for energy–burning.

Exercise such as walking kick–starts the body back into fat–burning mode. This is a slow process after extended periods of inactivity, but with repeated walks or other types of exercise, the fat-burning process becomes more efficient until eventually, the body burns more fat even while at rest or during sleep. When this happens, you have succeeded at speeding up your fat–burning metabolism. From this point onward, it will be easier for you to shed extra pounds.

The good news is that the more you walk or do other forms of exercise, the more fat you'll burn. The bad news is that if you stop exercising, your body will once again "forget" how to draw significant amounts of energy from fat deposits. The Cayce readings are clear about the importance of consistency: "Walking is the best exercise, but don't take this spasmodically. Have a regular time and do it, rain or shine!" (1968–9) Reading 308–13 is even more adamant about keeping up the momentum: " . . . regular exercise would be helpful, but don't start this and then do it for a day and then skip two or three days and then try it again; either do it regularly or don't begin . . ."

How much walking do you need to do in order to lose weight? Studies have shown that even if people do not change their diet, and provided they do not increase their daily food intake, a daily thirty-minute walk, taken on a regular basis, will prevent further weight gain. By increasing walking time and adjusting food intake, we cross the threshold and move from weight maintenance to weight loss. I emphasize "adjusting" rather than simply "reducing" food intake, because, as we have seen in the earlier chapters, weight loss is not strictly a question of calories or food quantity—it is the quality of the food that counts.

For reference purposes, the energy released from one pound of body fat is equal to about thirty-five hundred calories. If your objective is to lose one pound a week, you would need to burn some five hundred calories per day more than you did before you began your program. The average walker burns about one hundred calories per mile, which he or she walks in fifteen minutes. However, I do not recommend counting calories. As we have seen in the chapters on diet, not all calories are alike, and some foods actually help increase fat-burning metabolism. Remember, too, as explained above, that the more you exercise, the more fat you'll burn, so these numbers are mere guidelines.

Do you need to do all your daily walking at one time? Not necessarily. A recent study at Stanford University showed that, whether subjects exercised for thirty consecutive minutes or whether they divided their exercise time into three ten-minute segments a day, both groups increased their fitness level equally. So, if your schedule does not allow thirty minutes or more of uninterrupted walking every day, take heart. You can still benefit from shorter walks taken at intervals throughout the day. There may, in fact, be a benefit in dividing your walking time: a study reported in the September 2006 issue of *Hypertension* found that taking four short walks a day lowered blood pressure more than one long walk. For the purpose of kick-starting your body's fat-burning engine, however, longer periods of walking or other exercise have been shown to be more effective.

How do you keep up your daily walks in cold climes and inclement weather? If it's simply too cold or too wet to go outside, a treadmill may be the answer. Quality treadmills aren't cheap, but they may be an investment in your good health that you'll make frequent use of: research has shown that treadmills are the most used of the various types of indoor exercise equipment on the market. But even if you don't own a treadmill or don't want to invest in one, you can keep up some of your walking at home, for instance, by moving about while talking on the phone, walking up and down the stairs, or simply walking in one place. Even housework is a form of exercise and has been shown to provide many benefits.

Alternatively, during the winter months, you may temporarily wish to take up another indoor activity such as yoga or tai chi. The latter, an ancient Chinese system of exercise that focuses on slow, fluid movements, is particularly popular with seniors, who find that it gives them greater flexibility, better concentration, and a deep feeling of relaxation.

Whatever type of exercise you choose, it is important to keep the body moving on a regular basis to ensure that it continues to burn fat. Besides optimizing body weight, exercise has many other health benefits. It has been shown to protect against Alzheimer's disease and other forms of dementia, as well as cancer and depression. For instance, research reported in the December 2005 issue of *Medicine & Science in Sports & Exercise* showed that a single thirty-minute walk on a treadmill provided an emotional lift to patients who had been diagnosed with major depressive disorder.

Optimize your workout–take a deep breath

Our capacity to exercise is partially determined by our ability to breathe properly. Luckily, our breathing ability is also improved with exercise. Either way, breathing is vitally important if we want to be healthy, fit, and slim.

You might say that breathing is automatic, so why worry about it? After all, the body knows how to breathe. True, but there are factors that affect the quality of the breath you take and, with it, the amount of oxygen and nourishment that gets delivered to the cells.

Just pay attention to your breath for a moment. Do you inhale and exhale very quickly so that the air you draw in barely expands your chest? If so, take a deeper breath—inhale slowly through the nose, and draw the air deeply into the lower part of your lungs. See your abdomen expand with each incoming breath. Ah . . . that feels better! You can feel yourself coming more alive with each breath. This is because abdominal breathing is the most natural form of breathing.

You're likely seated while you read this book, but stand up for a minute. Straighten your spine and neck and take a slow, deep breath in through the nose. Now exhale gently, letting the air out through the nostrils. With your next incoming breath, lift up your arms as you breathe in, as much as feels comfortable. This allows you to take an even deeper breath. Deeper breathing allows more oxygen to reach deeply into the lungs, replacing stale air that has accumulated during periods of shallow breathing.

Because of poor breathing habits, most people use less than a third of their total lung capacity. This means that better breathing habits could more than double the amount of oxygen that reaches the lungs, the blood and, ultimately, the cells of the body. Increased oxygen means increased circulation and better detoxification and nourishment of all body cells—in short, a healthier you!

A breath of fresh air. When the body moves, it demands more oxygen. The more you exercise outdoors in the fresh air, the better. The Cayce readings recommend exercising our breath while walking: ". . . long walks morning and evening are well, as to the exercise; and when doing same breathe *deep* into the lungs." (272-8)

While walking outdoors, try these simple exercises: Stand erect and empty your lungs of air. Then slowly raise both arms to a horizontal position in front of you, breathing in gently and deeply while lifting your arms. Hold the breath for a moment. Continue lifting up your arms to an almost vertical position on each side of your head while continuing to inhale. As you raise your arms higher, draw in just a bit more air. Then gently lower your arms and breathe out slowly and completely. Repeat this exercise several times, mornings and evenings. Be persistent. Poor breathing habits have developed over a long period of time and it takes patience and perseverance to change them, but it is well worth the effort.

The increased oxygen supply that comes with exercise promotes mental clarity and brainpower. A study done at the University of Illinois in Urbana–Champaign showed that thirty minutes of moderately heavy to heavy running on a treadmill improved thinking ability and increased the speed of the decision–making process. On a smaller scale, but following the same principle, I try to get up and walk around whenever I've been sitting at my computer too long and find my thinking has slowed down or my memory fails me. It's usually not long before the answer to a question I held in my mind presents itself, or I remember what I had forgotten. Moving the body definitely helps move the mind!

Breathe away stress. Deeper and slower breathing is also the perfect antidote to stress. The fight-or-flight response, which most of us unconsciously adopt in response to a perceived stressor, causes muscles to contract and restricts breathing. By consciously altering the breathing pattern with deeper and slower breaths, it is possible to relax the entire nervous system in a relatively short time. The deeper the breath you take, the less often you will need to breathe. The average person breathes about sixteen times a minute. Those who are skilled in proper breathing breathe only five or six times a minute. The slower and deeper the breathing, the calmer the person. He or she is also far less likely to become breathless or fatigued.

You will notice that your posture plays a significant role in your ability to breathe well. When you are slouched in a chair or sofa, the rib cage compresses the lungs, making it difficult for them to fill with air. The more erect you sit or stand, the better your breathing capacity. Deep breathing, in turn, will strengthen muscles and help them work more efficiently, thus improving your posture. Even the internal organs receive a workout through proper breathing—the contracting and expanding diaphragm massages the kidneys, liver, stomach, and heart.

Breathing is the most vital of body functions. An improvement in breathing patterns and breathing capacity brings about an immediate improvement in all other body functions, including the metabolic rate. Breathing is the very foundation of life, and it enhances the body's ability to regenerate itself. Reading 2072-5 says, "Breath is the life-blood cleansing of the body . . . For, there are the needs for the combination of the gases as inhaled to act upon the purifying of the system." The next time you feel fatigued, listless, or lethargic, think of nature's instant energizer—take a deep breath!

Warm up to stretching

Professional athletes never miss an opportunity to stretch before getting into the action of a game or competition, and they keep their muscles warm and flexible with stretches while taking a break. But even if you aren't aiming for the Olympics, stretching the body and limbs is one of the best ways to stay flexible, keep your muscles tuned, and help you become a better fat-burner.

> **The stretching of the body; not in excess, but as a stretching of the arms, of the limbs—side, circular, forward, up, down. Not just as a setting-up exercise, but stretch the arms high above head—stretch the arms to the front—a swinging motion. Two to three minutes of this each day will make for wonders in the *feelings* and the activities of the body.**
>
> **684-1**

Stretching is also an important aspect of the disciplines used in the ancient Indian health system of yoga. Yogis keep their bodies amazingly flexible and youthful through stretching routines. Interestingly, several of the yoga postures prescribe stretches that resemble those recommended in the Cayce readings, which suggest, "Stretch the body as a cat would stretch. This is the best exercise to keep [the] body in proportion." (5271-1) In Oriental medicine, too, stretching of the meridian energy lines is regularly performed as part of a treatment or exercise program.

The Cayce readings recommend upward stretches as a morning exercise, such as the one outlined in reading 259-10: "Mornings—with plenty of air in the room, standing, stretch the body to the full height. Rise on toes and at the same time gently raise the arms, so that there is the exercise of the muscular forces as well as the raising of the structural portion of the body."

In general, the morning exercises recommended in the Cayce readings are designed to expand and draw the energy upward in the body in preparation for the day's activities, as shown in the following example, which also emphasizes the importance of coordinating the breath with the exercise movements:

> **Of morning, and upon arising especially (and don't sleep too late!)—and before dressing, so that the clothing is loose or the fewer the better—standing erect before an open window, breathe deeply; gradually raising hands *above* the head, and then with the circular motion of the body from**

the hips bend forward; breathing *in* (and through the nostrils) as the body rises on the toes—breathing very deep; *exhaling suddenly* through the *mouth*; *not* through the nasal passages. Take these for five to six minutes. Then as these progress, gradually *close* one of the nostrils (even if it's necessary to use the hand—but if it is closed with the left hand, raise the right hand; and when closing the right nostril with the right hand, then raise the left hand) *as* the breathing *in* is accomplished. Rise, and the circular motion of the body from the hips, and bending forward; *expelling* as the body reaches the lowest level in the bending towards the floor (expelling through the mouth, suddenly). See?

1523-2

Exercises to be done in the evening, on the other hand, are indicated to be more contractive, drawing the energy downward, with an emphasis on exercising the lower limbs, as explained in reading 2454-2: "When ready to retire, let the exercise preferably be for the lower limbs; this [is] a movement as of sitting on the floor and walking across, or swinging the limbs one in front of the other for three to four movements."

Eating for a great workout

During walking, stretching, and other forms of exercise, many changes occur in your body. Energy production is accelerated, muscle contractions increase, the heart beats faster to promote blood circulation, and the lungs work harder to accommodate increased oxygen requirements. This surge in metabolic activity requires extra energy, and you'll want to be sure to provide your body with all required nutrients for optimal energy and endurance. Let's review briefly the types of foods that will optimally support your exercise program.

High-performance muscle energy. Carbohydrates are the body's primary energy foods. They break down into glucose, which is stored as glycogen in muscle tissue and in the liver. During a workout, glycogen is quickly depleted from muscle cells and must be replenished. In your diet, emphasize whole, unrefined carbohydrates, such as vegetables and fruits, whole grains (brown rice, whole-grain bread and pasta), legumes, and nuts and seeds. Avoid refined and processed foods. Unrefined carbs provide a more sustained energy level by helping prevent blood glucose fluctuations.

High-powered protein. Protein plays an important role in tissue growth and repair, in maintaining optimal fluid balance, and in energy metabolism. Protein requirements are easily met in a natural whole-foods diet that includes eggs, dairy, and chicken or fish, if desired. Vegetarians can obtain protein from combinations of whole grains and legumes, nuts, or seeds. However, if a person's digestive system is not functioning optimally, protein assimilation from plant sources may be compromised.

Essential fats. Allow only natural fats, such as butter and unrefined vegetable oils (extra virgin olive oil, coconut oil, macadamia nut oil), in your diet. Avoid hydrogenated vegetable oils, which introduce harmful trans-fatty acids into the diet. Fish oil, taken in supplement form, can act as an aid to weight loss. A recent study demonstrated that study subjects who both took fish oil and exercised lost an average of 4.5 pounds over the course of the study without making changes in their diet. The fish oil appears to increase the body's fat-burning metabolism. Fish oil, in bottles as well as in capsule form, is available in natural food stores.

Rehydrate! Water is your greatest ally in protecting your body against fatigue and low energy! Water delivers oxygen, hormones, and nutrients to the cells. It helps lubricate joints and regulate body temperature. Drink plenty of pure water before, during, and after a workout. Sports drinks provide water along with electrolyte minerals, which are easily lost in sweating during exercise.

Timed energy release. Eat a meal high in unrefined carbohydrates two to three hours before beginning your workout. Half an hour before exercising, a snack of fresh or dried fruits, or a handful of nuts, provides a quick energy boost. Depending on the duration and intensity of your workout, replenish carbohydrates with a high-energy meal after exercising. Natural whole foods are the best choice for restoring energy levels, but if time and convenience dictate otherwise, energy bars formulated with all natural ingredients can help prevent muscle fatigue and exhaustion.

Be wise—don't compromise: providing your body with high–quality nutrients for your workout can make all the difference in the success of your exercise program.

Clearing cellulite naturally

A frequent beauty problem troubling those who carry extra pounds is cellulite, defined by *Webster's Medical Dictionary* as "lumpy fat found in the thighs, hips, and buttocks of some women." An estimated 80 percent of women experience symptoms of cellulite to varying degrees. The pharmaceutical and herbal health industries have cashed in on our desire to be rid of the condition by formulating numerous cellulite-reducing remedies, creams, and lotions.

Exercise such as walking, which stimulates fat–burning and promotes good circulation, is helpful in reducing cellulite. When the body becomes more efficient at dissolving fatty deposits and using them for energy, cellulite will naturally dissolve. There are several additional ways in which we can help the body get rid of this unsightly problem.

One of the conditions aggravating cellulite is an accumulation of toxins in the body. Any attempt to rid the body of poisons must first remove the most common cause of toxicity: constipation. Brisk sales of over–the–counter laxatives leave no doubt as to how widespread this condition is. However, most pharmaceutical laxatives, though temporarily effective, can irritate the colon, and habitual use often creates a dependence. For the support of regular bowel function and long–term prevention of constipation, it is preferable to increase fiber and ensure adequate liquid intake on a regular basis.

For quick relief of constipation, the husk of psyllium seeds is a gentle yet effective intestinal bulking agent that naturally stimulates a lazy colon into action. A tablespoonful in a large glass of water or juice, two or three times daily, can bring good results. For maximum effectiveness, plenty of liquid must be taken with the psyllium, which is highly absorbent. An alternative to psyllium is freshly ground flaxseed, high in mucilaginous fiber, which absorbs water and softens stools.

Naturally fermented, unpasteurized sauerkraut, homemade or commercially available in the refrigerated section of many natural food stores, is another excellent remedy due to the action of choline, which promotes peristaltic movement. The lactic acid in sauerkraut also helps recolonize the beneficial bacteria in the intestinal tract. And the old home remedy—soaked dried prunes—taken with the soaking water, is as effective today as it was in days past.

The Cayce apple diet. When proper bowel function is restored, we are in a much better position to tackle the next step toward cellular detoxification and the goal of dissolving cellulite. An excellent way to jump-start a cleansing program is with Edgar Cayce's apple diet, which we briefly discussed in chapter four. While on this regimen, only raw apples are eaten for two or three days—as many as desired. Plenty of water or unsweetened herbal tea should be taken in between. Before retiring on the last day, the apple diet is concluded by drinking half a cupful of olive oil (preferably extra-virgin, from the first pressing of the olives). Cayce suggested that the apple diet would cleanse toxins from the body and remove encrusted fecal matter in the colon.

For best results, the apple diet should be undertaken at a time of little or no stress. Choose a convenient time, such as a weekend, when you can move at your own pace without pressure from the demands of work or family life. Detoxifying can sometimes bring on fatigue, irritability, and headaches as toxins are flushed out of the tissues and into the bloodstream. This can often be eliminated by drinking more water.

Apples are high in pectin, a special type of absorbent fiber also found in grapes and lemons, which are likewise known for their detoxifying properties.

Colonic Irrigations. Another effective way for removing toxins from the body and encrusted fecal matter from the colon is colonic irrigation. The Cayce readings consistently emphasize the importance of keeping the colon clean and recommend colonics as an effective means to achieve this. The colon is the last collecting station in the passage that food takes through the body. Maintaining regular bowel function is important for colon health, as any fecal matter that remains in the colon can dry out and adhere to the colon walls. When the colon is thus impacted, it becomes difficult for the beneficial bacteria that normally populate the colon to survive. Unhealthy bacteria flourish instead, producing toxic by-products. Bowel toxicity has been associated with many health conditions, including arthritis, allergies, headaches, sinus congestion, and skin conditions.

Regular colonic irrigations help flush out encrusted fecal matter, toxins, and other impurities, resulting in greater energy and better overall health. Cayce reading 440-2 suggests that ". . . *every* one—everybody—should take an internal bath occasionally, as well as an external one. They would all be better off if they would!" The readings recommend colonics for numerous conditions, including arthritis, asthma, dermatitis, epilepsy, migraine headaches, and high blood pressure.

In a professional colonic, two tubes are inserted into the rectum through a speculum. The pure, lukewarm water is flushed in through one tube, and water and loosened fecal matter and impurities are flushed out through the other. During the process, the colon therapist performs a gentle massage of the client's abdomen, which encourages the flow of water and the cleansing process. A colonic irrigation is deeper than an enema. In fact, Cayce reading 3570-1 claims that "one colonic irrigation will be worth about four to six enemas."

External water therapy. Subjecting the body to alternating hot and cold water gushes or packs helps increase cellular circulation and thus detoxification and healing. Alternating hot and cold showers are an excellent way to benefit from this form of water therapy. After a warm bath or shower, simply turn on the cold water and remain there for as long as you can stand it, or move in and out of the cold stream. Although this might feel uncomfortable at first, it won't be long before you'll notice the energizing, refreshing effect of finishing your shower or bath with a cold water gush.

Once you have become used to this routine, you can begin alternating hot and cold showers. Begin with warm water, then cold, and then increase the temperature of the warm water to maximize comfort levels. Always finish with cold water, as this helps close the pores and tone the body. Although the water will feel cold against the skin, after toweling dry, you will feel warm and invigorated from the considerable increase in circulation.

Juice fasting. As we have seen in chapter four, another effective way for ridding the body of cellular toxins is through a juice fast. Most people in generally good health can benefit from going without solid food for one or more days. Juice fasts, especially those undertaken with freshly pressed fruit or vegetable juices, are easier on the body than strict water fasts. Fresh juices provide valuable vitamins, minerals, and enzymes that nourish the body while giving the digestive system a break from processing solids. The concentrated nutrients in juice further assist the cleansing process. In general, fruit juices have a stronger cleansing effect than vegetable juices, but the latter are preferred for those with blood sugar abnormalities. Fasts longer than three days should only be undertaken in consultation with a knowledgeable health professional.

Herbs for lymphatic cleansing. The lymph system is an intricate network of vessels and nodes along which flows the lymph, a milky-clear liquid that filters out waste products and delivers nutrients to body cells. Many health professionals consider cellulite to be caused by lymphatic congestion. The lymphatic system depends largely on muscular contraction, and thus exercise, to move the lymph along its pathways, especially lymph flowing to the peripheral areas of the body, including the cellulite-prone hips and thighs. Most forms of exercise, especially walking, running, cycling, or bouncing on a rebounder, are excellent for restoring lymph flow to these areas.

Certain herbs are known for improving lymphatic action. Echinacea, for instance, has a stimulating effect on the lymph system and has been shown to carry waste tissue away from areas of infection. Other effective herbs include cleavers, sarsaparilla, burdock, and garlic.

Edgar Cayce recommended a special herbal formulation consisting of several cleansing and detoxifying herbs, including sarsaparilla root, wild cherry bark, dog fennel, yellow dock root, dogwood bark, and prickly ash bark. This formula, marketed as *Herbal Tonic 545* by Baar Products (www.baar.com), is taken by the half-teaspoonful four times a day, before meals and before retiring. Cayce suggested it as a good spring tonic that would assist in clearing the entire system.

Detoxifying the liver. As the major organ responsible for detoxifying the body, the liver works continuously to break down and flush out toxic substances. However, an overload of toxins can leave the liver overworked and exhausted, causing symptoms such as fatigue, hormone imbalances, and weight gain.

Artichokes, or artichoke extract, are helpful if constipation is due to a sluggish liver, since they stimulate the production of bile, a natural laxative. Bitter herbs, taken in tincture form or as a tea, help relieve bloating, indigestion, and other intestinal complaints. These herbs include dandelion, milk thistle, and red clover. Formulations of bitter herbs are available in natural food stores or specialty pharmacies.

Chlorophyll, nature's powerful detoxifier, supports the cleansing process. It also helps activate enzymes, build blood, and promote tissue regeneration. Chlorophyll is abundantly present in deep green vegetables such as broccoli, kale, and chard. As a supplement, it is available in liquid form or in convenient tablets and capsules. Green food concentrates, such as those made from barley grass, wheat grass, and blue/green algae, also supply B vitamins and other nutrients required for optimal liver function. Vitamin C, taken in amounts of 1,000 to 6,000 mg a day, has excellent detoxifying action.

Castor oil packs applied abdominally over the liver area two or three times a week help draw toxins from the liver and promote lymphatic drainage. Prepare a bed or other flat surface where you can lie down comfortably. Cover the area with plastic sheeting (a large garbage bag does the trick well) and place an old towel on top on which you can lie down. Fold a cotton flannel cloth into several layers of thickness, and then soak it in castor oil. Place this over the liver area, and cover it with another plastic sheet to prevent soiling. Cover this with another towel, and then place a hot water bottle or an electric heating pad on top. Heat helps drive the oil through the skin into the tissues. Leave on for about an hour, during which time you can close your eyes and relax or meditate.

Afterward, wash the oil off your skin with a mixture of water and baking soda. (The commercial line of Cayce formulations also includes a special formula designed to help wash off the castor oil.) Don't discard your oil-soaked flannel cloth, as it can be reused many times. Keep it wrapped in plastic or in a suitable container for the next castor oil session. I keep mine folded in a glass pie shell covered with aluminum foil. Before the next use, I like to warm it up just a little bit in the oven so it will be warm on contact with the skin. Don't allow it to get hot, however; you don't want to burn the oil or your skin!

Castor oil packs were recommended in the Cayce readings for a variety of health conditions. By toning and strengthening the liver and lymphatic system, they are a tremendous aid in detoxification and rejuvenation of the body. Dr. William A. McGarey, who has clinically worked with castor oil packs and other medical suggestions from the Cayce readings for many decades, has summarized his extensive experiences with this remedy in his book *The Oil That Heals: A Physician's Successes with Castor Oil Treatments.*

Dry skin brushing. Dry skin brushing is another effective remedy for healing cellulite because it increases circulation, not only superficially, in the skin, but also throughout the entire body. It stimulates lymphatic activity, as well as cellular detoxification and renewal. Using a loofah or natural bristle brush, begin at the end of each limb and brush in a circular motion toward the center of the body and the heart. Avoid brushing areas that are inflamed or broken. Brushing before a shower or bath is best, since these further enhance circulation and allow dead and flaking skin cells to be rinsed away. Afterward, rub the skin with a firm towel and apply a high–quality natural skin lotion or oil, such as the following Cayce formulation:

Mix together 6 ounces peanut oil, 2 ounces olive oil, 2 ounces natural rose water, and 1 teaspoon dissolved lanolin, and shake well.

This formula is easy to prepare, but is best made in small quantities, because natural rose water spoils easily and, when combined with oils, promotes rancidity. A popular version of this formulation, which does not contain rose water but is prepared with vitamin E instead, is marketed as Olivae Skin Lotion by Baar Products (www.baar.com).

Additional anti-cellulite remedies. Hot compresses or poultices to the affected areas can also have a cellulite–reducing effect. Certain herbs, such as ivy or fenugreek, may be added for better results. Fenugreek seeds can also be taken internally to help prevent fatty deposits.

Deep tissue massage and lymphatic drainage massage are other effective methods for increasing circulation and breaking stubborn fatty deposits characteristic of cellulite. Lymphatic drainage massage is popular in Europe, where it has long been standard therapy in the treatment of cellulite.

Although certain commercial products on the market today promise quick success in curing this unsightly problem, it is important to recognize that a complex condition such as cellulite is best treated in a holistic manner. A multidimensional approach involving detoxification, optimal nutrition, exercise, and topical skin treatments is the surest way to improve the appearance of the skin and with it the health of the entire body.

10 Taming Stress

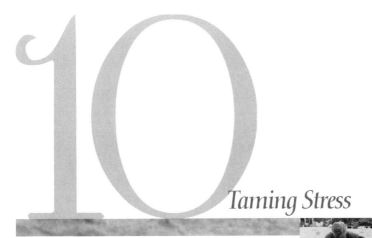

SEVERAL STUDIES HAVE SHOWN that if we're stressed, some of us tend to overeat. Our bodies also register other responses that range from increased levels of stress chemicals and higher cholesterol in the bloodstream to lack of sleep and depression. In fact, a study published by Statistics Canada in 2006 found that stress can be an important predictor in mortality. For optimal health and to keep our weight down, we need to learn to deal with stress in a positive and effective way.

Meditation is an ideal tool, freely available to all, for improving stress response and general well–being. Its benefits range from greater mental clarity and physical relaxation to relief from fatigue and the numerous improvements in physical health it has been shown to produce. Several studies have also reported that meditation effectively lowers blood pressure in both adults and children.

The Cayce readings emphasize the importance of regular periods of meditation, saying that everyone will eventually have to learn how to meditate. Meditation can be defined as the practice of quieting our physical bodies and our minds, and focusing inward and on the mind of God. It has often been said that meditation is listening to God, while prayer is talking to God.

There are many systems of meditation, some involving a mantra or affirmation, while others focus on breathing or employ chants to quiet the mind. A simple way to begin meditating is to find a comfortable place to sit down—either a chair or a pillow on the floor. It is important that when you are seated, you are able to keep your spine straight without discomfort. Put your hands loosely in your lap and close your eyes. Now breathe deeply into your lungs; breathe in and out slowly and deeply several times until you begin to feel relaxed.

Next, focus your mind on an inspiring thought, affirmation, or mantra that appeals to you. If you can't think of anything, you may wish to find a biblical verse or a line from a spiritual song or poem. Some people like to play soft spiritual music or chants in the background. Perhaps you would just like to visualize a high-vibration color, such as pure white, gold, or purple. When you have made your choice, keep this affirmation or visualization *in your heart as well as in your mind.* It is important that you not only *think* about it, but that you also *feel it.* When you can feel it without needing to think about it, stay with this feeling for as long as you are comfortable.

Throughout the process, you may find yourself becoming distracted by various thoughts that are causing your mind to wander. Don't be concerned about this phenomenon, as it is perfectly normal. With regular practice, your meditations will become deeper and you will be less easily distracted.

When you close your meditation session, give thanks for the experience, ask for healing for yourself and others, and send out the meditative feeling and healing you have experienced into the world and to other people. Some people like to open their hands and allow the energy to flow through them and be released outward. Then slowly open your eyes and bring your attention back to the room and your environment.

The A.R.E. has published many books on the practice and benefits of meditation. Visit EdgarCayce.org for more information on the various meditation tools and courses available.

Meditation is an important practice for connecting with our spiritual essence and experiencing our connection with God and all of creation. Many studies have shown the enormous benefits of a regular spiritual practice. Meditation helps us discover the purpose for which we have entered the world and to identify and remove the blockages that prevent us from unfolding our spiritual potential. Our full spiritual potential includes perfect health and our perfect weight. We need only to ask and be willing to receive the blessing.

Stress-free eating

It is never a good idea to eat when you feel stressed. Conditions of worry, tiredness, and strain within the body must be considered as an influence that combines with the effect of foods. The next reading touches on this in greater detail:

> . . . we would find at times there are various conditions and various foods that produce, under the stress and strain of activity, a varied effect . . .
>
> When the body is under stress or strain by being tired, overactive, and then would eat heavy foods—as cabbage boiled with meat—these would produce acidity; yet cabbage without the meats would produce an alkaline reaction under the same conditions! The same would be true if there were fried foods such as fried potatoes eaten, when there is a little cold or the body has gotten exceedingly cold or damp, these would produce (if fried) an acid, and become hard upon the system; while the same taken as mashed or as roasted with other foods would react differently. **1411-2**

It is better under such conditions to abstain from food, or at least from a heavier meal, until the stress has been put aside and one is able to once again digest and assimilate foods properly. Tension, fear, and worry inhibit the secretion of digestive juices, which results in incomplete digestion and poor assimilation. It is best to eat in a relaxed, peaceful atmosphere.

It is also important during a meal to be conscious of the act of eating, which includes chewing all foods well. The better we chew our food, the less work the digestive system has in breaking it down further. While chewing, it helps to become aware of the taste of the food and to visualize what we want the body to do with it. Our consciousness while eating has an effect on how the food is processed.

> **That thou eatest, see it *doing* that *thou* would *have* it do. Now there is often considered as to why do those of either the vegetable, mineral, or combination compounds, have different effects under different conditions? It is the *consciousness* of the *individual body!* Give one a dose of clear *water*, with the impression that it will act as salts—how often will it act in that manner?**   **341-31**

If you want your food to go to work in building a healthier, slimmer you, your next meal is the time to visualize this outcome!

Get your sleep to lose your weight

One might assume that sleep, a time of relative inactivity for the body, would be associated more with weight gain than weight loss. Yet, in recent years, a growing body of research points to the opposite—indicating a direct relationship between sleep deprivation and weight gain.

In the same measure that the number of obese people has grown in the industrialized world, there has been a decrease in the number of hours that we spend sleeping every night. In a large study reported at a meeting of the North American Association for the Study of Obesity in 2004, involving eighteen thousand adults, the less study subjects slept, the greater their chances were of being obese. Those who got less than four hours of sleep per night were 73 percent more likely to be obese than those who slept seven to nine hours. Among those who slept five hours per night, the risk was 50 percent greater, while those sleeping six hours increased their risk by 23 percent. Similar results were obtained in 2006 in a study conducted at Case Western Reserve University. Results of the sixteen-year study involving 68,183 middle-aged women showed that women who slept five hours or less each night were 32 percent more likely to gain a significant amount of weight and 15 percent more likely to become obese than women who slept seven hours each night. The weight was gained even though the women who slept less also ate less, and it was demonstrated that both diet and exercise were not a factor in the weight gain of the women who slept less.

What could cause such certain but seemingly counterintuitive values in the relationship between sleep loss and weight gain? One of the theories discussed is based on evidence that there's a connection between sleep and the various neural pathways that regulate food intake. Losing sleep seems to raise levels of hormones associated with appetite control and eating behavior. People who are sleep-deprived have reduced values of leptin, a hormone through which the brain senses that satiety levels have been reached and that there's no more need for food. Sleep-deprived individuals, however, have a 28 percent increase in the hormone ghrelin, which triggers hunger. On average, those who consistently sleep five hours or less per night have been shown to have 14.9 percent more ghrelin and 15.5 percent less leptin than those who sleep eight hours per night.

To be sure, we sleep less not only as individuals—as a society, too, we have embraced the 24/7 lifestyle as if it were the most natural thing in the world. We shop at twenty-four-hour supermarkets, business centers, and restaurants. We ignore nature's light/dark cycles each time we turn on the lights in our homes and offices after it gets dark. We run our TVs, radios, and computers around the clock and expect all systems to be up and functioning without interruption. By going against nature's rhythms, we have unknowingly set ourselves up for trouble, as our lack of sleep is reflected in our expanding waistlines. Clearly, our attempts at autonomy in the sleep/wake cycle have backfired.

A similar pattern of less sleep/more weight gain has also been observed in children. A study published in the November 2006 issue of *Archives of Disease in Childhood* reports on the growing body of research that suggests that cutting down on sleep may lead to metabolic changes that contribute to obesity, diabetes, and heart disease in children as well as in adults. Because our lives have become so busy, we have turned into an entire society of tired, sleep-deprived adults and kids.

For those of us who are serious about losing extra pounds, then, one thing should become clear: We need to make sleep a priority, along with diet and exercise. The Cayce readings emphasize the need for adequate sleep, often suggesting that early-to-bed/early-to-rise is the pattern that would best serve our sleep needs and natural body rhythms. Cayce referred to sleep as the sixth sense, which "acts from the nervous system." (849-20) He explained that "there is an active force within each individual that functions in the manner of a sense when the body-physical is in sleep . . ." (5754-2) It appears that this active force also helps the sleeper to be a better fat-burner.

Planning better sleep

Although most sleep is lost because we are too busy for it, even when we do make the time, we are not always successful at falling or staying asleep. Resorting to pharmaceutical sleeping aids in such situations is a bad choice. Sleeping pills are addictive, requiring ever larger doses to become effective. In addition, they actually suppress a period of the sleep cycle known as REM sleep. REM is an acronym for Rapid Eye Movement, which occurs during this deep-sleep phase when the large muscles in the body are relaxed, but brain activity is high, and the eyes can be seen moving rapidly underneath closed eyelids. It is during REM sleep that most dreams occur.

REM phases alternate with non-REM (NREM) sleep, when brain activity registers slower wave patterns. During a typical night, the sleeper moves through several cycles of REM sleep. The amount of REM sleep we get is correlated with the amount of mental and emotional stress we experience during the day. A lack of REM sleep causes feelings of nervousness and stress during the day, which signals that REM sleep, and the dreams that occur during it, are an essential stress-reduction mechanism.

An increasing body of research also indicates that sleep helps consolidate memories, thus promoting effective learning.

Certain neurotransmitters play an important role in sleep regulation. The best known of these is serotonin, which is essential for promoting relaxation and sleep. Another chemical, the hormone melatonin, which is produced by the pineal gland, plays an important role in promoting good sleep. Melatonin is regulated by the natural cycle of light and darkness. The use of indoor lights and insufficient exposure to natural sunlight during the day suppress melatonin secretion, resulting in varying degrees of sleep disruption.

Digestive problems are a major reason why many people are unable to sleep. Eating the last meal of the day no later than three hours before going to bed helps prevent digestive discomforts during the night. Avoid eating greasy, fried foods and combinations of large amounts of protein and starch at the same meal. These are difficult to digest and often cause bloating and gas. Avoid or reduce the consumption of caffeinated beverages, especially in the late afternoon or evening. Coffee, black tea, and colas all contain caffeine. Staying up too late or working the late-evening shift can itself cause digestive problems, as a study reported in the 2004 issue of the *American Journal of Industrial Medicine* showed.

A number of herbal remedies are highly effective in promoting sleep naturally. Valerian root is one of the most popular herbs for relieving insomnia and anxiety. Several research studies have confirmed the ability of valerian to gently sedate the central nervous system and promote restful sleep without risking addiction.

Essential oil of lavender has a relaxing effect on the nervous system and has been shown in several studies to help those who have difficulty sleeping. Lavender oil placed in an aromatic diffuser or oil burner in the bedroom allows the fragrant molecules to be released into the air. Alternatively, a few drops of the oil may be sprinkled on a pillow or handkerchief placed close to the face.

Other sleep-promoting herbs include camomile, linden flower, catnip, and skullcap. The Cayce readings recommend an old folk remedy for insomnia, a glass of hot milk sweetened with honey, to be taken at bedtime. The easily digested simple sugars in honey promote the conversion of the amino acid tryptophan, found in milk (as well as in turkey, gourds, and nuts), to the important sleep chemical serotonin.

A bedtime snack of calcium-rich foods, such as almonds, dates, figs, or sesame seeds, also helps produce a relaxed state in the body. Edgar Cayce's Mummy Food, discussed in chapter eight, is an ideal bedtime snack.

Keep the room that you sleep in dark. Darkness promotes the

production of the sleep chemical melatonin. Your bedroom should be well ventilated and cool, but not too cold. Low–frequency fields generated by electrical appliances can interfere with sleep, and such devices are best unplugged if they are located close to the bed.

Getting a good night's sleep will do more than just keep us awake during the day—it will also keep us slim.

Chapter Summary

Getting Started on Your Cayce Diet and Health Program

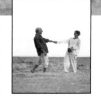

NOW THAT YOU HAVE READ the earlier chapters in this book, you may ask, Well, all of this sounds pretty good, but how do I actually apply all these things, and how can I make them a part of my daily routine without being overwhelmed?

It is true that too many pieces of information can seem overwhelming when not condensed and distilled into a usable formula. And yet, it is important to have a solid understanding of the reasons behind the formula if you want to feel comfortable applying it.

In this section, I have tried to summarize the steps recommended in each of the chapters outlining the five principles of healthy eating (chapters three through seven), as well as the additional steps explained in chapters eight through ten. I hope this will make them easier to remember and implement, while at the same time enabling you to refer back to the appropriate chapter for a more detailed discussion, if required.

Healthy Eating Principle No. 1
Indulge in Water   (chapter three)

Helpful tips for increasing your water intake:

- Make it a habit to drink one or two large glasses of water first thing after getting up in the morning. Add a few drops of freshly squeezed lemon or lime juice, or a combination of both. This will kick–start your metabolism, help remove toxins from your system, and give you a head start on your daily water intake.
- Make it a habit to drink a large glass of water half an hour before each meal.
- Whenever you feel hungry, drink a large glass of water before you reach for something to eat. Then wait ten minutes to see if you are still hungry. If not, you were thirsty rather than hungry. If you still feel hungry, you will likely eat less than you would have without drinking water first, and you will then digest and assimilate your food better.
- Whenever you feel thirsty, drink water before reaching for any other drink. After you have satisfied your thirst with water, feel free to drink juices or other naturally flavored beverages in moderation. But use only water to quench your thirst.
- Make it a habit to carry water with you wherever you go, whether you are walking, cycling, or driving. If you wish to avoid carrying disposable plastic bottles, consider investing in a stainless steel thermos bottle or other durable container in which to transport your water.
- If your work is sedentary, make it a habit to keep a glass or bottle of water on your desk so that you can take frequent sips from it. If you move around a lot in your work, try to find a convenient way of keeping water accessible while you work.

Healthy Eating Principle No. 2
Favor Veggies and Fruits   (chapter four)

Helpful tips for increasing your intake of veggies and fruits:

- Aim to eat one entirely raw meal each day, such as a large salad for lunch. If this is not possible, eat a small salad with lunch and dinner.
- Keep snacks of sliced veggies or fruits in your fridge, to grab when

you're on the run or too busy to cook a healthy meal.
- Think of vegetables as the major component of each meal instead of considering them as a side dish.
- Keep canned or frozen veggies and fruits in your pantry or freezer. Although fresh foods are always best, canned or frozen veggies and fruits are better than none.
- Drink diluted grape juice (two parts juice to one part water) half an hour before each meal. This helps promote weight loss by changing the way the body processes starches and sweets.
- Invest in good cookbooks featuring vegetables, and take advantage of free recipe cards being offered in many grocery stores. This helps take the monotony out of eating and introduces you to new ideas for incorporating more veggies and fruits in your diet.

Healthy Eating Principle No. 3
Prioritize for Protein   (chapter five)
Helpful tips for maximizing protein power:
- Eat regular servings of protein foods throughout the day to maintain energy levels.
- Keep healthy protein snacks such as cheese wedges and yogurt in your refrigerator.
- Leftover cooked chicken can be stored in the fridge for up to two days. Slice it up as a handy snack, or toss it in salads for added protein power.
- If you are a vegetarian, remember to combine grains and legumes, nuts, or seeds for complete protein.
- Remember that a protein meal keeps you feeling full longer.
- While protein is important, you only need a small quantity of it at each meal. You don't need to eat a whole chicken breast, for instance. Enjoyed in smaller amounts, protein is more easily digested and assimilated.

Healthy Eating Principle No. 4
Keep Starches in Check   (chapter six)
Helpful tips for cutting down on starches:
- Do not eat two starches at any one meal. For instance, if you eat

potatoes, do not eat rice at the same meal. Eat vegetables instead.
- Commit to eating only whole grains and baked products; avoid all foods made with refined flour and rice.
- Choose breads made with sourdough for added nutrition and assimilation.
- Try some of the alternative grains discussed in chapter six.
- If you wish to eat dessert, try custard, ice cream, or fruit rather than starchy pies or cake.

Healthy Eating Principle No. 5
Banish Fake Fats   (chapter seven)
Helpful tips for eliminating bad fats from your diet:
- Read all labels and avoid foods made with hydrogenated oils and vegetable shortenings.
- Beware of dangerous fat substitutes in products labeled "fat-free."
- Use butter or extra-virgin olive oil for cooking. Remember, these natural healthy fats are important for proper metabolic function.
- Use coconut oil or butter for baking.
- Purchase only cold-pressed oils stored in dark glass bottles.
- Avoid refined vegetable oils found on supermarket shelves.

Treats to Slim Down With   (chapter eight)
Helpful tips for incorporating healthier snacks into your diet:
- Keep healthy snacks based on whole foods in your home and at your place of work, so you won't be tempted to buy junk food when hunger strikes.
- If you can't resist snacks such as potato chips, for instance, look for those that are baked rather than fried.
- Transfer snack items from large bags into smaller, portion-sized containers. When a snack-attack strikes, eat only the measured portion. Some restraint is necessary for successful weight management.

Get Physical—Burn Fat Fast   (chapter nine)
Helpful tips for increasing physical activity:
- Walk, rather than take the car, to any destination that allows you to

do so. Allow yourself the extra time this requires. This time is not lost to you. It will return to you in the added energy that will result if you keep up your walks on a daily basis.

- Join a walking group in your neighborhood. This will help keep you inspired and entertained while exercising.
- Take the stairs, rather than the elevator, whenever possible. Make it a habit, for instance, to use the elevator only if you need to go higher than three flights of stairs (or any number that you can comfortably manage).
- Try to think of a sport that inspires you, and then find a creative way of incorporating it into your lifestyle.
- Whatever you do—remember to breathe deeply. This will increase energy levels and keep you moving.

Taming Stress (chapter ten)

Helpful tips for taming stress and getting better sleep:

- Set aside time for meditation daily. Meditation helps you cope with stress effectively.
- Don't eat when you're stressed, worried, or upset. Wait until you have relaxed and are able to digest and assimilate your food better.
- Be conscious of the taste and texture of your food while eating. Chew all foods well. Visualize in what ways you want your body to use the foods for fuel.
- Make sleep a priority. Determine an optimal bedtime for you that allows you to get sufficient sleep, and then adhere to it as closely as possible.
- Do not eat anything other than relaxing snacks, such as almonds, bananas, yogurt, or milk, within three hours prior to going to bed. Going to bed on a very full stomach impairs the quality of your sleep.
- If possible, make it a habit to go to bed early and get up early, rather than staying up late and sleeping in late. Your body is designed to sleep when it is dark and to be active and awake in daylight. When you are out of sync with this natural rhythm, your sleep/wake cycle is disturbed and the function of your endocrine system will be compromised. A healthy endocrine system will help

you keep your weight down.

- Establish a regular period for meditation prior to going to sleep. This will help you to relax and tune in with your higher self and purpose. Your sleep will subsequently be deeper and more refreshing.

- If you are tempted to ignore your body's need for sleep because there are more important things to do, remember that fewer hours of sleep is associated with greater weight gain. Don't deprive your body of one of the most effortless ways to keep your weight down!

Should you take supplements?

Originally intended to fill in the gap for those suffering from specific vitamin or mineral deficiencies, food supplements have evolved into a class all their own. Touching on alchemical dimensions, they claim to hold the secrets to everything from the fountain of youth to limitless brain power—all natural, of course, and free of side effects. Weight loss is no exception. An impressive lineup of nutraceutical products promises to help you shed unwanted pounds, clear up your cellulite, and rejuvenate saggy skin following weight loss. The question is, do you believe these claims?

My advice would be to keep your cool. Use supplements for the purpose for which they were designed: to *supplement* the diet. First, eat the best possible natural whole-foods diet, and then worry about supplements. Above all, don't skimp on food quality because you rely on supplements. No supplement will completely make up for a poor diet. Nature has put important phytochemicals in food that science has yet to discover.

With that said, food supplements do have a role to play in a natural foods diet. Soil erosion, as well as aggressive commercial farming methods, has depleted our agricultural soils of minerals, and if these nutrients are not in the soil, they will not be in our food. My preferred approach to food supplementation is one that relies on food–sourced ingredients, that is to say, supplements made from concentrations of superfoods, in which nature has supplied the formula. These types of supplements are the most bioavailable to the body. Fortunately, today, the supplements industry is offering an increasing range of such food–based supplements.

The Cayce readings offer an interesting perspective on supplements, suggesting that they be taken for a period of time, then suspended, then resumed, to ensure that the body not become lazy in its efforts to synthesize nutrients from foods:

> **All such properties that add to the system are more efficacious if they are given for periods, left off for periods and begun again. For if the system comes to rely upon such influences wholly, it ceases to produce the vitamins even though the food values may be kept normally balanced.**
>
> **And it's much better that these be produced in the body from the normal development than supplied mechanically; for nature is much better yet than science!**   **759-13**

Some of the readings also explain that supplements should not be taken until the eliminative pathways in the body are functioning effectively, because supplements would otherwise only increase any existing conditions. A woman asked in a reading if she should take vitamins, and was given this response:

> **These are well to be taken when there is not a tie-up in the eliminations. When eliminations are set up, take same. But if these are taken under the stress of the lack of functioning of the eliminating forces of the body, these produce more hindrances than helpfulness. They are as boosters—and if you boost a pain–do you relieve it, or get more pain? 307-21**

So, first get your digestive system in shape by drinking lots of water, eating fiber–rich whole foods, getting regular exercise, applying castor oil packs, and keeping toxins out of your system—and then take supplements periodically if necessary.

The Cayce readings themselves offer formulas for certain herbal combinations that are said to have specific cleansing and rejuvenating effects on the body. The following is a partial list of those formulations that would be of interest to those wishing to optimize digestive power and weight loss:[4]

- **A digestive tonic** that was said to be "good for everyone as a spring tonic" and to "assist in clarifying the whole system," containing several cleansing and tonifying herbs, including sarsaparilla root, wild cherry bark, dog fennel, yellow dock root, dogwood bark, and prickly ash bark
- **An intestinal tonic** combining wild ginseng, wild ginger, tincture of stilingia, and elixir of lactated pepsin, in a grain alcohol base
- **A revitalizing and energizing tonic** that was said to rejuvenate the glandular system and stimulate digestion, made from elixir of lactated pepsin, liver extract, black snake root, ginseng, and Atomidine–an aqueous solution of iodine from iodine trichloride (Atomidine is also available individually and can be taken to stimulate the glandular system.)

A tea prepared from the herb American saffron (*carthamus tinctorius*) is frequently recommended in the readings to balance the digestive system, promote detoxification, and achieve better coordination between the organs of assimilation and elimination. Cayce reading 5545-1 advises: "Just before the *meals* are taken, that of a *mild* tea of Saffron should be able to coat the whole of the stomach proper. This will aid digestion."

For general nutritional support, you may want to consider taking a quality green–foods concentrate or bee pollen, which is the male germ cell of flowers, herbs, and tree blossoms that bees collect as their food. Bee pollen is considered a complete survival food, containing all essential amino acids, vitamins, enzymes, and fatty acids.

For natural endocrine support, sea kelp in powder or tablet form is often very helpful. Kelp is a rich source of minerals, particularly iodine, which supports the healthy function of the thyroid and rejuvenates the entire glandular system.

---

[4] To order these and other Cayce products mentioned in this book, visit baar.com in the United States, and EdgarCayceCanada.com in Canada.

To address specific nutritional deficiencies or dietary concerns, please consult a qualified nutritionist or other natural health practitioner.

Hippocrates said, "Let food be your medicine, and your medicine your food." In the twenty-first century, one of our greatest challenges is to keep our food supply safe, healthy, and free of toxic substances. Only natural whole foods can provide the physical sustenance for the body and help it return to its proper weight.

Affirmation for weight loss

Prayer and affirmations help reinforce our intention and enlist divine intervention in the manifestation of our intent. Read and say this affirmation daily, or write down your intention in your own words and refer to it frequently to align your thoughts and actions and infuse them with divine help. Ask and you shall receive.

> Today, I become conscious of my true nature
> As a child of God—and a co-creator with Him.
> Today, I choose to nourish and recreate
> My body temple in the perfect image of my Creator.
> I select healthy foods that make it easy
> To find my perfect weight.
> The way is clear, for my body is my friend
> And supports my intention for its optimal health.
> Today, I take the next step on the road
> To perfect health and perfect weight.
> I am fully supported by the Divine
> And I give thanks for this perfect support.
> Amen

Know that all strength, all healing of every nature is the changing of the vibrations from within—the attuning of the divine within the living tissue of a body to Creative Energies.
1967-1

Recipes Section

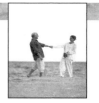

THIS SECTION CONTAINS A SELECTION OF RECIPES for meals with wholesome ingredients that will support you in your efforts to gain greater health and achieve weight loss.

Several of these recipes come with compliments of my dear friend and colleague Andrea Lemieux, whose culinary skills far surpass my own. Others originated from my own kitchen.

Some of the recipes are modeled strictly on the Cayce diet, others lean toward the Mediterranean diet, and some take inspiration from Middle Eastern or East Indian cuisine. All use natural ingredients and cooking methods. The Cayce readings, as we have seen, do not recommend cooking foods with any type of fat or oil, even though either butter or olive oil may be added after cooking. Unrefined sea salt and other seasonings, too, are to be added after cooking. Each food is gently cooked on its own and then combined with other foods at the meal. This is unquestionably the purest and healthiest way to cook, and this is the method most compatible with the suggestions from the Cayce readings.

However, it does make the presentation of recipes somewhat monotonous. Better said, perhaps, it makes recipes unnecessary because most foods are prepared in the same manner and then combined. However, to offer greater variety and a wider range of flavors and aroma, several of the recipes included do use both olive oil and butter, as well as natural herbs and spices, in the cooking process.

I trust you will enjoy both types of recipes as you work on creating a healthier and slimmer you!

Breakfast Dishes

Basic Continental Breakfast
SERVES 1
$1/2$ grapefruit
1 slice whole-grain toast (whole wheat, spelt, or kamut), buttered
1 egg, poached or soft-boiled
Black coffee or tea, or natural coffee substitute

Oatmeal Porridge
SERVES 1
$1/2$ cup steel-cut or rolled oats
$1/2$ cup water
1 teaspoon yogurt
$1/8$ teaspoon unrefined sea salt
$1/2$ cup water
1 tablespoon maple syrup, sucanat, date sugar, or unpasteurized honey

Mix oats and salt with $1/2$ cup water and yogurt; cover, and let stand at room temperature overnight or for as long as 24 hours. Bring one additional half cup of water to a boil. Add soaked oats; reduce heat, cover, and simmer 7 to 10 minutes.

Sweeten with maple syrup, Sucanat, date sugar, or unpasteurized honey. Serve with black coffee or tea, or a natural coffee substitute, if desired.

Scrambled Eggs with Bacon

SERVES 1

2 eggs
1 strip crisp, organic bacon, chopped fine
1 tablespoon butter

Melt butter in hot skillet. Combine bacon with eggs and scramble in skillet.

Optional: 1 slice whole-grain toast. Glass of freshly squeezed orange juice. Black coffee or tea, or natural coffee substitute

Edgar Cayce's Mummy Food

SERVES 4

1 cup Black Mission figs
1 cup dates (seeded)
1^1/2 quarts water
1 cup cornmeal
1 cup half-and-half cream (optional)

Combine figs, dates, and cornmeal with water and cook for about 30 minutes. May be served hot or cold, with or without cream.

Creamy Rice Cereal

SERVES 1

1 cup cooked brown rice
^{3}/4 cup milk
^{1}/2 teaspoon vanilla
^{1}/4 teaspoon cinnamon

Add all ingredients together. Heat if desired. Add more milk or cream to taste or to adjust texture.

Banana Yogurt Granola

SERVES 1

1 banana

1/2 cup yogurt

1 tablespoon granola

Slice banana. Mix with yogurt and granola.

Optional: Black coffee or tea, herbal tea, or coffee substitute

Salads
. . . .

Cheesy Summer Salad

SERVES 2

1 romaine lettuce heart

1 stalk celery

1 vine-ripened tomato, chopped or cut into small wedges

1/4 purple onion, thinly sliced

2 tablespoons fresh parsley, chopped

1/4 cup cheddar cheese (ideally, raw-milk cheese), grated

Dressing:

3 tablespoons extra-virgin olive oil

2 tablespoons fresh lemon juice

1/2 teaspoon unrefined granulated sea salt

1/8 teaspoon gelatin powder (optional)

Wash and chop lettuce, celery, tomato, onion, and parsley. Toss together in salad bowl.

In a small mixing dish, combine olive oil, lemon juice, sea salt, and gelatin powder. Mix well. Pour over salad mixture. Sprinkle with grated cheddar cheese.

Red and green salad

SERVES 2

1 stalk red leaf lettuce

Several sprigs watercress

1 medium carrot, grated

1/2 beet root, grated

1/2 cucumber, peeled and diced

Wash and chop lettuce and watercress. Add prepared carrot, beet root, and cucumber. Serve with your favorite salad dressing or with olive oil, lemon juice (or wine vinegar), and unrefined sea salt.

Tabbouleh

SERVES 2

1 cup water
1/4 teaspoon salt
1 cup dry bulgur wheat
1 cup tomatoes, finely diced
1 cup cucumber, seeded and finely diced
1/2 cup purple onion, finely chopped
1 bunch parsley, finely chopped
1 tablespoon extra-virgin olive oil
1 tablespoon basil
1/3 cup fresh lemon juice
1/2 cup yogurt

Add salt to water and bring to a boil. Pour bulgur into boiling water, cover, and turn off the heat. Let stand 20 minutes, then place in fridge to cool. Mix with next 7 ingredients.

Serve with yogurt.

Chinese Green Bean Salad

SERVES 4

1 pound fresh, organic green beans
1 tablespoon fresh ginger root, finely chopped

Dressing:

4 teaspoons dry mustard powder
1 tablespoon cold water
2 tablespoons tamari soy sauce
3 tablespoons freshly squeezed lemon juice
2 teaspoons extra-virgin olive oil

Trim and slice the beans crosswise, into 1-inch lengths. Place in appropriately sized sheet of Patapar paper; fold and steep the pouch in rapidly boiling water for about 15 minutes. Remove beans from pouch. Drain juice into a glass container, then mix with the dressing ingredients and toss with the ginger root and green beans.

Fruit Salad

SERVES 2

1 large orange
2 cups grapes
1 cup strawberries in season
1/2 fresh pineapple, chopped
2 bananas, chopped
1/2 tablespoon freshly squeezed lemon juice
1/2 tablespoon freshly squeezed lime juice
Fresh mint
1 tablespoon maple syrup, if desired

Peel orange and cut into chunks; wash grapes and remove from stem; wash and chop strawberries. Combine all fruits and sprinkle with lemon and lime juice. Garnish with fresh mint. If desired, pour maple syrup over mixture.

Salad Dressings

Note: The Cayce readings advise against vinegar, due to its acidity. Small amounts of pure wine vinegar, which is less acidic, are permitted for healthy individuals.

Garlic-Mustard Vinaigrette

3 tablespoons wine vinegar
1/4 teaspoon unrefined sea salt
1 tablespoon whole-grain mustard
2 cloves garlic
1/3 cup extra-virgin olive oil

Place the vinegar, salt, and mustard in a bowl. Peel the garlic and squeeze it through a garlic press into the vinegar mixture. Whisk; add the oil in a slow trickle, and continue whisking until dressing thickens.

Tamari Vinaigrette

3/4 cup extra-virgin olive oil
2 tablespoons whole-grain mustard
1 tablespoon freshly squeezed lemon juice

3 to 4 tablespoons wine vinegar
1/2 teaspoon unrefined sea salt
1 tablespoon tamari soy sauce

Place all the ingredients in a screw-top jar or small bowl, and shake or whisk to blend well.

Olive-Mustard Dressing

1/2 cup extra-virgin olive oil
1/4 cup wine vinegar
1 heaping tablespoon whole-grain mustard

Combine all the ingredients in a small bowl or screw-top jar, and whisk or shake well to blend.

Mustard Cream Vinaigrette

3 tablespoons wine vinegar
2 tablespoons umeboshi vinegar
2 teaspoons whole-grain mustard
1/2 cup extra-virgin olive oil
1 tablespoon tahini (sesame butter)

Mix the vinegars and mustard together in a small bowl. Whisk in the oil very slowly until the dressing emulsifies. Then whisk in the tahini. Alternatively, combine all the vinaigrette ingredients in a blender or food processor and process for 30 seconds.

Herbal Vinaigrette

3/4 cup olive oil
1/4 cup wine vinegar
2 green onions, chopped
2 sprigs fresh parsley or 1 1/2 teaspoons dried
1 clove garlic, minced
1 tablespoon freshly squeezed lemon juice
1 teaspoon unrefined sea salt
1/2 teaspoon each: basil, marjoram, anise seed, and dill weed
1/8 teaspoon cayenne pepper

Combine all ingredients in blender, and blend for two minutes or until smooth.

Yogurt-Garlic Dressing
1 cup plain yogurt
2 teaspoons olive oil
2 cloves garlic, finely minced
2 tablespoons freshly squeezed lemon juice

Whisk all ingredients together in a screw-top jar. Close lid and shake vigorously.

Avocado Dressing
$1/2$ cup olive oil
2 ripe, medium avocados
4 teaspoons fresh, chopped parsley
1 teaspoon fresh lemon juice
$1/4$ teaspoon unrefined sea salt
Dash of powdered sea kelp
Cayenne pepper to taste

Whisk all ingredients together in screw-top jar. Close lid and shake vigorously.

Soups . . . .

Chicken Noodle Soup with Vegetables
SERVES 4
2 cups chicken stock (prepared by boiling chicken bones, including back
and neck bones, for at least two hours, then strained)
1 onion, chopped
2 cloves garlic, chopped
3 carrots, chopped
4 ribs celery, chopped
$1/2$ cup soup noodles
1 tablespoon unrefined sea salt
1 tablespoon Herbamare herbal salt

*Prepare chicken stock. Cook onion, garlic, carrots, and celery in 6 cups water
until soft. Add chicken stock and noodles. Bring to boil and cook until noodles
are done. Add sea salt and herbal salt.*

Cool-off Gazpacho

SERVES 4

1 onion, chopped
3 cloves garlic, chopped
6 vine-ripened tomatoes, peeled if desired
1 cucumber, peeled and chopped
1 green pepper, seeded and quartered
2 cups tomato juice
2 tablespoons dried basil or fresh
1/2 cup fresh lemon juice
1/4 cup extra-virgin olive oil

Puree all ingredients in a blender or food processor. Serve chilled.

Serve with two slices of crisp bread, spread with 4 tablespoons cottage cheese.

Potato Zucchini Puree

SERVES 5

2 white onions, quartered
5 medium-sized, yellow-flesh potatoes, quartered
3 medium-sized green zucchini, cut into large chunks
2 tablespoons butter
1 tablespoon unrefined sea salt
1 tablespoon Herbamare herbal salt
15 whole-grain crackers
5 tablespoons cream cheese

In a large saucepan, bring to boil three cups of water. Add onions, potatoes, and zucchini and cook over medium heat 20-25 minutes. Add butter and seasonings; stir well. Blend all ingredients in blender to desired creamy texture. Serve with whole-grain crackers and cream cheese.

Broccoli-Carrot Cream Soup

SERVES 4

1 tablespoon butter
1 medium onion, chopped
1 large carrot, chopped
2 tablespoons whole wheat flour

3 cups water
2 vegetable or chicken bouillon cubes
1 bunch broccoli, chopped
1 cup milk
Dash of cayenne pepper

In a large saucepan, melt the butter over medium heat. Add chopped onion and carrot; sauté 5 minutes. Remove saucepan from heat and whisk in the flour. Add water and bouillon cubes; bring to boil. Add chopped broccoli. Reduce heat and simmer, uncovered, 5 to 7 minutes or until broccoli is tender.

In a blender or food processor, puree soup in batches until smooth; return to saucepan. Add milk and cayenne. Heat through, but avoid boiling.

Broccoli-Leek Soup

SERVES 4

4 cups chicken broth (prepare by boiling chicken bones, including back and neck bones, for at least two hours, then strain)
1 tablespoon extra-virgin olive oil or butter
1 medium onion, chopped
1 leek, well rinsed and chopped coarsely
1 small celery root, approximately 2 oz (50 grams), peeled and cut into very small pieces
1 bunch broccoli, chopped, including some of the stalks, peeled
1 teaspoon unrefined sea salt
Cayenne pepper to taste

Prepare chicken stock.

Heat oil or butter in a soup pot on medium heat. Sauté onion, leek, and celery root, stirring for about 10 minutes.

Add broccoli and pour chicken broth over vegetables. Add more broth or water to cover vegetables, if necessary. Bring to a light boil, reduce heat; cover and simmer until broccoli is tender, 8-10 minutes.

Transfer soup in batches to a blender or food processor and process. Return to pot; season with salt and cayenne. Heat through and serve.

Note: Can be frozen.

Hearty Brown Lentil Soup

SERVES 6

1 1/2 to 2 cups brown lentils
4 cups water
2 tablespoons extra-virgin olive oil
1/2 teaspoon each: garlic powder, dried basil, and paprika
1/4 teaspoon each: cumin powder and oregano
2 large onions, chopped
2 garlic cloves, finely diced
2 ribs celery, diced
1 carrot, diced
1 potato, cut into small chunks
3 tomatoes, diced (use canned tomatoes when tomatoes are not in season)
8 to 10 cups water or vegetable stock, depending on desired thickness of soup
4 tablespoons tamari
2 teaspoons unrefined sea salt, or to taste

Sort, rinse, and drain the lentils. Cook them in about 4 cups of water for 30 minutes.

While the lentils are cooking, heat the oil in a large saucepan. Add garlic powder and spices, except for tamari and sea salt, and sauté for 2-3 minutes. Gradually add onions, garlic, celery, carrot, potato, and tomatoes, sautéing them in the oil and spices. If the tomatoes are not juicy enough, add water to desired consistency.

After the lentils have cooked for 30 minutes, add them to the vegetable mixture; add the water or vegetable stock. Bring to a boil and simmer for an additional 30-45 minutes. Add sea salt and tamari toward the end of cooking. Correct seasoning to taste.

Carrot-Ginger Soup

SERVES 4 TO 6

8 cups vegetable stock
3 cups carrots, peeled and sliced
1 medium potato, peeled and sliced

2 teaspoons extra-virgin olive oil
1 medium onion, chopped
3 tablespoons fresh ginger root, peeled and finely chopped
Unrefined sea salt to taste
Dash of nutmeg
Fresh parsley or cilantro, chopped (optional)

Place the carrots and potato in a pot with the vegetable stock. Bring to a boil; cover, reduce heat, and boil gently until the vegetables are tender, about 30-45 minutes. Heat the olive oil in a skillet; add the onion and ginger, and sauté, stirring, just until onion is translucent. Remove from heat. When carrots and potato are tender, add onion and ginger to the pot, and cook together for 5 minutes.

Puree the soup in batches in a blender or food processor. Add salt to taste, and flavor with the nutmeg. Serve plain or garnished with chopped, fresh parsley or cilantro.

Pureed Potato Soup with Arugula

SERVES 6

1 tablespoon butter
4 leeks, washed and chopped
2 cloves garlic, minced
3 large, unpeeled potatoes, washed and diced
4 cups chicken stock or water
$1/4$ teaspoon cayenne pepper
$1/8$ teaspoon dried thyme
1 tablespoon unrefined sea salt (or to taste)
1 bunch arugula, washed and coarsely chopped

In a large saucepan, melt butter; add leeks and garlic; and cook for about 5 minutes. Add potatoes and stir mixture well; add stock or water, cayenne, and thyme. Bring to a boil; reduce heat and simmer 30 minutes or until potatoes are cooked through; add sea salt.

Blend soup in blender in batches and return to saucepan. Add chopped arugula; heat just until wilted. Adjust seasoning to taste.

Fish Dishes

Wild-caught Pacific Salmon Steak with Butter and Lemon Sauce

SERVES 1

1/2 wild-caught Pacific salmon steak
2 tablespoons butter
1/4 cup fresh lemon juice
2 cups kale, chopped
1/2 cup cauliflower florets
1/2 cup green beans, chopped
1/2 cup brown basmati rice
1 cup water
1/2 teaspoon unrefined sea salt, divided

Wash rice and place in water with 1/4 teaspoon sea salt. Bring to boil. Reduce temperature and simmer for 40 minutes.

Preheat oven to 375°. Place salmon steak on baking dish and dot with 1 tablespoon butter. Bake for 20-25 minutes.

Add chopped vegetables and cook in steamer or patapar paper for 15 minutes.

Before serving, pour lemon juice over salmon. Sprinkle with remaining 1/4 teaspoon salt. Add remaining tablespoon butter to vegetables and rice. Serve immediately.

Parchment Red Snapper and Vegetable Bake

SERVES 1

1 red snapper fillet
1 tablespoon butter, melted
1 tablespoon lemon juice
1 tablespoon tamari soy sauce
1/2 cup carrots, chopped
1/2 cup acorn squash, chopped
1 cup kale, chopped
2 tablespoons extra-virgin olive oil
1/2 cup parsley, chopped
Unrefined sea salt and Herbamare herbal salt to taste

Preheat oven to 350°. Rinse fish with cold water. Place in center of parchment paper. Combine melted butter with lemon juice and tamari soy sauce; pour over fish. Fold paper over the fish, leaving a "hem" around the edge. Secure with pin or paper clip. Bake for 25-30 minutes. Cut paper and slide out fish onto a plate; pour juices over the fish.

Mix carrots, squash, and kale with olive oil and arrange in baking dish. Sprinkle with unrefined sea salt and Herbamare herbal salt. Bake alongside the fish for 25-30 minutes, then remove from oven.

Sprinkle fish and vegetables with chopped parsley.

Baked Halibut and Vegetables

SERVES 4

Note: You can substitute other types of fish for the halibut, and you can use fillets instead of steaks.

4 halibut steaks
Water
1 small zucchini, cut into 1/4-inch slices
1 tomato, chopped
1 cup snow peas, trimmed
2 green onions, chopped
1/2 teaspoon dried basil or 2 teaspoons minced, fresh dill
1/4 teaspoon unrefined sea salt

Preheat oven to 350°.

Place the fish in a single layer in a baking dish. Add just enough water to cover the bottom of the dish, about 1/4 cup.

Cover and bake at 350° for 5 minutes. Remove from the oven and arrange the zucchini, tomato, snow peas, and green onions around the fish. Sprinkle with the basil or dill, and salt. Cover and bake for 10 to 15 minutes more, or until the fish flakes easily when tested with a fork.

Broiled Salmon Steaks

SERVES 2

2 salmon steaks
2 tablespoons freshly squeezed lemon juice

1 tablespoon tamari
1 teaspoon fresh ginger root, minced or grated
1 large garlic clove, minced

Mix together the lemon juice, tamari, ginger, and garlic. Pour over the salmon steaks, and marinate in the refrigerator for 20 minutes, turning the steaks over after 10 minutes.

Reserve marinade and place the salmon on a lightly buttered broiler pan. Broil for 10 minutes per inch of thickness, measured at the thickest part, or until the salmon flakes easily when tested with a fork. Turn the steaks over halfway through the cooking time, basting with reserved marinade. Serve hot or cold.

Poultry Dishes

Baked chicken leg and vegetables

SERVES 1

1 medium-sized chicken leg, skin on
1 medium-sized potato, including skin, cubed
1 large carrot, or two small carrots, chopped
1/4 head cauliflower florets
1 cup Brussels sprouts, halved
2 tablespoons fresh parsley, chopped
1 tablespoon butter for seasoning vegetables (optional)
Unrefined sea salt to taste

Preheat oven to 350°. Place chicken leg in a glass baking tray or casserole dish. Sprinkle sea salt on the skin. Bake in oven for 40 minutes. While chicken is baking, chop all vegetables separately. Place on separate squares of Patapar or strong parchment paper, then form into a pouch. Use cotton string to tie each pouch together at the top.

Fill a large saucepan with 2 inches of water. Bring to a boil. Place the three parchment paper pouches containing the chopped veggies in the saucepan. Allow to cook for 15 minutes. When serving the vegetables, pour the juice that has collected in the pouch over the vegetables. (Alternatively, steam the chopped vegetables in a steamer.) Serve together with the baked chicken leg, from which the skin has been removed. Season to taste with butter and unrefined sea salt.

Chicken with Lemon and Herbs

SERVES 2

2 chicken breast halves
1 garlic clove, minced
1 teaspoon extra-virgin olive oil or butter
1 tablespoon freshly squeezed lemon juice
1 tablespoon water
1/2 teaspoon oregano
1/2 teaspoon basil
Pinch unrefined sea salt

Preheat oven to 350°. Place the chicken in a baking dish. Combine the remaining ingredients and pour over chicken. Bake uncovered, basting occasionally, for 30 to 35 minutes for boneless, 40 to 45 minutes for bone in, or until chicken is no longer pink inside.

Garlic Chicken

SERVES 4

4 chicken legs, skin on
1 tablespoon butter
7-8 cloves garlic, thinly sliced
2/3 cup white wine
1 1/2 teaspoons unrefined sea salt

Preheat oven to 400°.

Melt butter in large, ovenproof pot over medium heat. Add chicken legs and brown very, very lightly on both sides. Pile chicken to one side in pot.

Add garlic and sauté for three minutes; do not let burn. Arrange chicken legs in pot, turning them to coat well in the garlic. Add salt. Pour wine over the chicken.

Cover pot and place in oven. Bake at 400° for 40 minutes. Serve with brown rice and a green salad and/or other vegetables.

Roast Chicken

SERVES 2

Note: A whole chicken can be roasted for two people; you will have leftovers for another meal.

One whole chicken
2 tablespoons butter
Dried thyme
Unrefined sea salt
1 small carrot, sliced
1 stalk celery, sliced
White wine

Preheat the oven to 350°.

Wash the chicken inside and out under the tap. Dry with paper towels. Salt the inside of the chicken, then put the sliced carrot and celery into the cavity for flavoring.

Put the chicken in a shallow roasting pan. (It is not necessary to truss the chicken.)

Melt the butter with dried thyme. Use more butter and thyme as desired. Spread the butter/thyme mixture all over the chicken with a pastry brush.

Pour a little white wine into the bottom of the pan, and put pan in the oven. Baste with more butter/thyme after 15 minutes. Roast for a total of 25 minutes per pound (generally 1 1/4 to 1 1/2 hours).

Note: You can also roast potatoes, pearl onions, and/or carrots with the chicken. Put potatoes (in their jackets) in cold water to cover, bring to a boil, and cook for 10 to 15 minutes, until barely tender. Drain and put in the roast pan with the chicken for the last hour. Turn in the drippings and sprinkle with salt and pepper. Carrots or onions should also be steamed or sautéed slightly before roasting.

Poached Chicken Breasts

SERVES 2

2 cups (approximately) homemade chicken broth
2 teaspoons fresh rosemary, chopped
1 garlic clove, quartered
2 boneless, skinless chicken breast halves

Fill a deep skillet or a saucepan with just enough chicken broth to cover the chicken. Add the rosemary and garlic and bring just to a boil. Reduce heat to a very gentle simmer and, using tongs or a slotted spatula, add the chicken. Cover and simmer for 12 to 15 minutes, until the chicken is no longer pink inside, turning the chicken over after 6 minutes. *Remove the chicken and drain before serving. Discard the poaching liquid and other ingredients. Makes 2 servings.*

Note: *If you don't have chicken broth on hand, use water instead and add about 1 tablespoon of freshly squeezed lemon juice.*

Vegetable Dishes

Govinda's Vegetable Cheese Casserole

SERVES 2 TO 3

1 potato, cut into small cubes
1 small onion, chopped
2 carrots, chopped into small cubes
2 zucchini, chopped
1 cup broccoli florets
2 cups green cabbage, shredded
1 cup cauliflower florets
2 cups grated cheddar cheese
1 teaspoon Herbamare herbal salt

Preheat oven to 325°. Mix all vegetables and herbal salt together in a medium-sized casserole dish. Sprinkle with grated cheddar cheese. Bake 45 minutes.

Zucchini Toss

SERVES 4

2 tablespoons extra-virgin olive or butter
2 garlic cloves, peeled and finely chopped
$1/2$ teaspoon dried basil
4 medium zucchini, sliced into $1/2$-inch rounds
Dash of unrefined sea salt
Dash of cayenne pepper

Heat the oil or butter in a large frying pan over medium-high heat. Add the garlic and basil and cook for about 30 seconds, or until the garlic begins to sizzle. Add the zucchini and stir. Turn down the heat to medium low, and cook for about 3 minutes for crisp zucchini; for softer zucchini, cook for 5 minutes, or until they can easily be pierced with a fork. Season with salt and cayenne.

Tomato-Zucchini Stew

SERVES 2 TO 3

1-2 teaspoons butter
1 onion, chopped
4 tomatoes, chopped
1 large zucchini, chopped
1 green pepper, chopped
Oregano and basil to taste
Pinch unrefined sea salt

Melt the butter; sauté onions until soft. Add tomatoes, zucchini, green pepper, oregano, basil, and salt. Simmer one-half hour.

Asparagus Omelet

SERVES 2

$1/2$ pound asparagus, trimmed
Salted water
2 tablespoons butter, divided
1 garlic clove, minced
$1/2$ pound mushrooms, sliced
4 eggs, lightly beaten
$1/8$ cup milk
$1/2$ teaspoon unrefined sea salt
$1/4$ teaspoon dried basil, crushed, or $3/4$ teaspoon fresh

Cut asparagus spears into 1-inch pieces; cook in boiling, salted water until tender, about 2-4 minutes. Drain.

Melt 1 tablespoon butter in 8-inch skillet. Sauté garlic and mushrooms until done and moisture has evaporated. Remove from pan; keep warm.

In a small bowl, combine eggs, milk, salt, and basil. Melt remaining butter in skillet until foamy, swirling it around in pan to coat evenly. When hot enough that a drop of water sizzles when dropped in, pour in egg mixture. Tip pan so eggs coat skillet evenly. As eggs cook, periodically lift up cooked edges, tilt pan, and let uncooked egg run underneath.

When eggs are cooked, but surface is still shiny, place asparagus and mushrooms on one side; slide out of pan, folding side without vegetables over top. Serve immediately.

Asian Cabbage Stir-Fry

SERVES 6

1 tablespoon butter
1 tablespoon olive oil
2 tablespoons fresh ginger, chopped, or $1/2$ teaspoon dried
1 medium onion, chopped
1 tablespoon sesame seeds
1 small head green cabbage, or $1/2$ medium
2 tablespoons tamari
$1/8$ teaspoon cayenne pepper

In a large frying pan, melt butter and combine with olive oil. Stir in ginger, onions, and sesame seeds and cook for 2 minutes. Add cabbage and cook, stirring occasionally, for about 5 minutes or until tender crisp.

While cabbage is cooking, combine remaining ingredients. Add to cooked cabbage in pan and heat through.

Desserts

Strawberries 'n Cream

SERVES 1

$1/2$ cup sliced strawberries
$1/2$ cup half-and-half cream

Pour cream over strawberries and serve.

Summer Berry Frappé

SERVES 3

1 cup fresh or frozen strawberries
$1/2$ cup fresh or frozen blueberries
$1/2$ cup fresh or frozen raspberries
1 large banana or 2 small, peeled
1 cup water

1 tablespoon freshly squeezed lemon juice
1 tablespoon freshly squeezed lime juice

*Combine all ingredients in blender, and blend for two minutes or until smooth.
Serve in short, plump cups.*

Note: This tastes best when at least one of the ingredients is frozen.

Baked Apples

MAKES 4 TO 6 SERVINGS

4 to 6 apples, 1 per person (spy apples are the best variety for baking)
1 cup raisins
$1/2$ cup walnuts or pecans, chopped and lightly toasted at 300° for 10 minutes
2 tablespoons tahini
Juice and grated rind of 1 organic orange (free of pesticides, wax, and food coloring)
$1/4$ teaspoon cinnamon
$1/2$ teaspoon vanilla extract (optional)
Pinch of unrefined sea salt

Preheat oven to 375°.

Core the apples and peel a 1-inch strip around center of apple, or pierce skin with a fork to prevent bursting. Place apples in baking dish or glass pie pan.

Mix remaining ingredients, except orange juice, in a bowl. Fill center of each apple.

Pour orange juice into baking dish around apples.

Cover with foil; bake at 375° for 30 minutes. Test with fork to see if tender. Continue baking if needed.

Variations:

- *Substitute chopped dates or other dried fruit for raisins.*
- *Add a pinch of powdered ginger or allspice.*

Ginger Almond Pears

MAKES 5 SERVINGS

5 firm, ripe pears, Bartlett or Anjou
3 cups organic apple cider
2 teaspoons fresh ginger root, finely chopped
3 tablespoons arrowroot starch
1/2 teaspoon pure almond extract
Unrefined sea salt to taste

Peel the pears, quarter them lengthwise, and core. Slice pears thinly and place in a saucepan with the apple cider and ginger root. Add a pinch of salt. Bring to a boil, reduce heat, and simmer until pears are tender, about 15 minutes. Dissolve arrowroot starch in 1/3 cup cold water and add to the simmering pears, stirring, until the sauce is thick and clear. Remove from heat and stir in almond extract. Serve warm or cold.

Poached Apples with Whipped Cream

MAKES 4 SERVINGS

3/4 cup pure maple syrup
1 cup pure water
16 whole cloves
4 large, firm cooking apples (spy apples are best), peeled and cored
1/2 cup chilled, heavy cream, stiffly whipped

In a heavy 3- to 4-quart saucepan, bring the maple syrup and water to a boil over high heat.

Firmly insert 4 cloves in a ring around the top of each apple.

Place the apples side by side in the pan; baste with the syrup. Reduce the heat to low, and cover. Basting occasionally, simmer for 15 minutes, or until the apples are tender.

Remove from heat to cool in the syrup.

To serve, transfer the apples to individual dessert dishes. Pile whipped cream in the center of each apple, and pour over it a tablespoon of the syrup.

Internet Resources

For updates and resources connected with this book, visit
www.edgarcaycediet.com

A.R.E. Clinic, Phoenix, Arizona
www.areclinic.org

Baar Products Inc.
www.baar.com

Edgar Cayce Canada
www.edgarcaycecanada.com

Meridian Institute, spirit–mind–body research
www.meridianinstitute.com

Dr. John O. A. Pagano's psoriasis healing
www.psoriasis-healing.com

Dr. F. Batmanghelidj's water cure
www.watercure.com

Masaru Emoto's work with water crystals
www.masaru-emoto.net

Weston A. Price Foundation
www.westonaprice.org

The Green Guide—Smart Shopper's Fish Picks
www.thegreenguide.com/gg/pdf/fishchartissue97.pdf

U.S. Environmental Protection Agency's Fish Advisories
www.epa.gov/waterscience/fish/

Index

A

Acid/alkaline balance, *see also* pH
Balance
acid- and alkaline-forming foods, 12
major premise of Cayce diet, 11–14
measured on pH scale, 12

Acrylamide, *see also* Cooking methods
created in foods cooked at high
temperatures, 39

Alkaline diet, *see also* pH Balance
alkaline-forming foods, 12
alkaline reserve, 12
major premise of Cayce diet, 11–13

Almonds:
disease-preventing properties, 87

Apple diet, 42, 105
for detoxification, 105

Apples, *see also* Fruits; Apple diet
nutritional benefits, 41–42
pectin, 105

Artichoke:
liver stimulant, 108

Arugula:
nutrients occurring in, 24

B

Batmanghelidj, F., Dr., 19

Beef, *see also* Meat; Protein
beef juice, 59
restricted in Cayce diet, 59

Blueberries, *see also* Fruits
anticarcinogenic properties, 42
antioxidants occurring in, 42

Breakfast, 78–79
eggs, reducing hunger, 61. *See also* Eggs

importance of eating, 78
recipes, 129–131
recommendations for, 79

Breathing, 98–100
abdominal, 13
deep breathing:
as part of cleansing regimen, 32
improves posture, 100
with exercise, 98–100

Broccoli, 32–33. *See also* Vegetables,
cruciferous
anticarcinogenic properties, 33
anti-inflammatory properties, 33
nutritional benefits, 33

Brussels Sprouts, *see also* Vegetables,
cruciferous
nutritional benefits, 33

Butter, 82–83. *See also* Fats
easily digested, 83
from pasture-fed cows, 81

C

Cabbage, *see also* Vegetables, cruciferous
protects against stomach ulcers, 34

Canning:
of fruits and vegetables, 48–49
nutrient content affected by,
48–49
preferred for tomatoes if not vine-
ripened, 49

Carbohydrates, *see also* Glycemic index;
Grains; Starches
whole vs. refined, 72–73

Castor oil packs:
as part of cleansing regimen, 32,
108–109
effective for weight-loss, xiii

Cayce, Edgar:
  life and work of, ix–xiv

Cayce diet:
  alkalinity enhanced by, 11
  definition, xiii
  weight loss achieved with, xiii

Cellulite:
  therapies for, 104–109

Cheese:
  how to store, 63–64
  varieties recommended, 63

Chicken, *see* Poultry

Chlorophyll, *see also* Vegetables, green
  leafy
  detoxifying properties, 108

Chocolate, 91–92

Citrus fruits, 42–43
  cleansing properties, 43
  for prevention of colds, 43
  grapefruit:
    promoting weight loss, 43

Clinton, Bill, President:
  campaign against childhood
    obesity, 2

Cod liver oil, 81

Cola syrup:
  for medicinal purposes, 21

Collards, *see also* Vegetables, cruciferous
  nutritional benefits of, 33–34

Colonic irrigation, 105–106

Combining foods, *see* Food combining

Cooking methods, 39–41
  acrylamide:
    created in foods cooked at high
      temperatures, 39
  cookware:
    nontoxic, 40
  deep-frying:

not recommended, 41
frying:
  not recommended, 13, 41
lycopene:
  made bioavailable through
    cooking, 39
microwave oven:
  not recommended, 40
Patapar parchment method, 39–40
steaming, 40

Cookware, *see also* Cooking methods
  nontoxic, 40

Cruciferous vegetables, *see* Vegetables,
  cruciferous

Curly endive:
  nutritional benefits, 24–25

D

Dandelion greens:
  nutritional benefits, 25

Drying:
  of fruits and vegetables, 50–51

Dry skin brushing, *see* Skin brushing

E

Edgar Cayce's Mummy Food, 90–91
  as spiritual food, 90
  origins of, 89
  recipe, 91

Eggs, 59–61
  cholesterol in:
    not cause of heart disease, 60
    repair substance, 60
  egg replacers, *see also* Protein
    not recommended, 61
  how to store, 61
  methods of preparation, 60
  nutritional value, 59–60
  reducing hunger, 61
  supporting weight loss efforts, 60

Emoto, Masaru, Dr., 22

Enzymes:
  digestive:
    produced by pancreas, 27
  in raw foods:
    destroyed by heat, 28
    preserve digestive enzymes, 27
  supplementary, 29

Escarole:
  nutritional benefits, 24–25

Exercise, 93–104. *See also* Walking
  consistency required, 96
  how to achieve, 122–123
  disease-preventing qualities of, 98
  for morning and evening, 101–102
  importance of, 94
  increases breakdown of fat cells, 93
  nutrition for, 102–104
  stretching, 100–102

F

Fasting, *see* Fruit juices, fasts with

Fats, 15–16, 80–87. *See also* Oils
  adjusting diet to healthy fats, 122
  butter, 81, 82–83
  oils safe for cooking, 41
  olive oil, 83–85. *See also* Olive Oil
  omega-3 fats, 86
  required for nutrient assimilation, 26

Fermenting:
  of vegetables with lactic acid
    bacteria, 51

Fiber, *see also* Glycemic index; Grains
  benefits intestinal tract, 71–72
  optimal daily intake, 72

Fish, 66–68. *See also* Meat; Protein
  contamination of, 66–67
  methods of preparation, 59
  recipes, 140–142
  recommended in Cayce diet, 59, 66
  safety information references, 67
  storage information, 67–68

Food combining:
  citrus fruits and cereals:

not recommended, 79
  proteins and starches:
    restriction advised, 63
  sugars and starches:
    restriction advised, 77

Fowl, 64–65. *See also* Meat; Protein
  preparation methods, 59
  recommended in Cayce diet, 59
  turkey and wild turkey, 65

Freezing:
  of fruits and vegetables, 49–50
    nutrient content affected by, 50

Fried foods, *see also* Cooking methods
  not recommended, 13, 41

Fruit juices, fresh, 29–32. *See also* Fruits,
  Grape juice
  alkaline-forming, 13, 29
  easily assimilated, 29
  fasts with, 31–32, 106–107
  recipes, 30–31
  types of extractors, 29–30

Fruits, 41–45. *See also* Apples; Fruit juices,
  fresh; Grapes
  benefits of, 14–15
  boosting intake:
    to prevent weight gain, 41
  canning to preserve, 48–49
  citrus fruits, *see also* Citrus fruits
    nutritional benefits, 42–43
  dried, as healthy snack, 88–89
  drying to preserve, 50–51
  freezing to preserve, 49–50
  how to store, 46–47
  locally grown:
    benefits of, 51–52
  organically grown, *see also*
    Organically grown foods
    benefits, 53–57
    higher nutrient content, 54–55
  pectin, 105

G

Game, *see also* Fowl; Meat; Protein
  recommended in Cayce diet, 59
  wild turkey, 65

Glycemic index, 72–74
    foods ranking low on:
        promoting weight loss, 73

Grains, *see also* Glycemic index; Starches
    wheat alternatives, 74–75
    whole:
        fiber occurring in, 71–72
        how to prepare, 73
        nutritional value, 70–74
        sour-leavening, 73

Grapefruit, *see also* Citrus fruits; Fruits
    promoting weight loss, 43

Grape juice, *see also* Fruit juices; Grapes
    diluted, to combat obesity, 44
    recommended for weight loss, 11

Grapes, *see also* Fruits; Grape juice
    antioxidant properties, 43
    cleansing properties, 43
    resveratrol in red grapes:
        anti–obesity properties, 44–45

H

Herbal tonics (Cayce formulations), 126

Honey, 77–78. *See also* Sweeteners

Huckabee, Mike, Arkansas governor:
    campaign against childhood
        obesity, 2

I

Inulin:
    in Jerusalem artichokes, 34. *See also*
        Jerusalem artichokes

J

Jerusalem artichokes, 34–36
    blood sugar stabilizer, 34–35
    how to prepare, 35
    inulin, 34
    seasonal availability, 35

K

Kale, *see also* Vegetables, cruciferous
    nutritional benefits, 33–34

Kelp, 38, 126. *See also* Sea vegetables
    endocrine–balancing properties, 38
    salt substitute, 38

L

Lactic acid bacteria, *see also* Sauerkraut;
    Yogurt
    juices fermented with, 31
    milks fermented with, 62
    vegetables fermented with, 51

Lamb, *see also* Meat; Protein
    methods of preparation, 59

Lemieux, Andrea, 128

Lettuce:
    leaf lettuce preferable to head
        lettuce, 24

Litmus paper:
    to test pH balance, 13

Liver:
    detoxification, 107–109
    stressed by toxic chemicals, 31
    supported by fasts, 31

Lycopene:
    made bioavailable through cooking,
        39

Lymphatic cleansing, 107

M

MacDonald, Catherine, xiii

Massage, therapeutic:
    as part of cleansing regimen, 32

McGarey, William A., Dr., xii, 109

Meat, *see also* Protein
 frying not recommended, 59
 preparation methods, 59
 processed meat:
  not recommended, 66
 red meat:
  restricted in Cayce diet, 59

Meditation:
 alkaline influence of, 13

Mediterranean diet:
 associated with disease prevention,
 23

Microwave oven, *see also* Cooking
 methods
 not recommended for cooking, 40

Milk:
 fermented milks, 62. *See also* Yogurt
 homogenization, 62
 how to store, 63–64
 low-fat:
  not recommended, 62
 pasteurization, 61–62
 skim:
  not recommended, 62

Miso soup:
 alkaline-forming, 13

Mummy Food, *see* Edgar Cayce's
 Mummy Food

N

Nutritional supplements, *see*
 Supplements, nutritional

Nuts, 86–87
 as healthy snack, 89
 healthy oils occurring in, 86–87

O

Obesity:
 children affected by, 2
 financial burden created by, 3–4

global threat, 3–4
 health problems created by, 5
 income levels of people affected by,
 3–4
 life expectancy jeopardized by, 2
 number of Americans affected, 1

Oils, *see also* Fats
 coconut:
  source of medium–chain
   triglycerides, 86
 evening primrose, 86
 hydrogenated:
  not recommended, 85
 olive oil, 41, 83–85. *See also* Olive oil
 pumpkin, 86
 walnut, 86

Olive oil, 83–85. *See also* Oils
 anti–inflammatory effects, 83
 for acid reflux, 84
 safe for cooking, 41

Organically grown foods, 53–57
 cost considerations of, 56–57
 crop rotation in organic farming, 53
 for optimal nutrition, 12–13, 53–57
 for personal and planetary health,
  55–56
 higher nutrient content, 54–55
 organically farmed livestock, 54
 pesticides used in conventional
  farming, 53–57

Overweight:
 European statistics, 2–3
 malnutrition of individuals affected,
  4
 number of Americans affected, 1
 risk for diabetes, 1
 WHO global predictions, 2

P

Parsley:
 nutritional benefits, 25

Patapar parchment, *see also* Cooking
 methods
 cooking in, 39–40

Pesticides, *see* Organically grown foods

pH Balance, *see also* Acid/alkaline
 balance; Alkaline diet
 how to measure, 13
 influenced by diet and lifestyle, 13

pH Paper
 to test pH balance, 13

Physical activity, *see* Exercise

Pottenger, Francis, 81
 research with processed foods, 81

Poultry:
 recipes, 142–145
 recommended in Cayce diet, 64–66

Prayer:
 promoting alkalinity, 13

Price, Weston A., Dr., 80–81

Processed foods, *see also* Grains; Meat
 not recommended, 13
 promoting ill health, 80–82

Protein:
 complete, 58
 from plant foods, 58–59
 important for energy metabolism,
  103
 optimizing intake, 121
 requirements for, 15
 stimulates glucagon production, 59

R

Raw foods, 24–26. *See also* Enzymes, in
 raw foods; Salad(s)
 importance of eating, 26

Red wine:
 glass per day, recommended, 13, 44
 resveratrol occurring in:
  anti-obesity properties of, 44–
   45

Reilly, Harold J., Dr., xii

S

Salad(s):
 dressings:
  recipes 133–135
 recipes, 131–133
 vegetables for use in, 24–26

Salt:
 whole vs. refined, 75–76

Sauerkraut, 31, 51. *See also* Lactic acid
 bacteria

Schmidt, James, xiii

Sea vegetables, 36–39
 kelp, 38, 126
 weight-loss promoting compound
  in, 36

Skin brushing:
 as part of cleansing regimen, 32, 109

Sleep, 114–118
 how to improve, 116–118
 lack of, related to weight gain, 114–
  116

Snacks, 88–92
 as meal substitutes, 88
 Mummy Food. *See* Edgar Cayce's
  Mummy Food
 selecting healthy snacks, 122

Soft drinks:
 artificial sweeteners in, 21
 associated with weight gain, 21

Soup recipes, 135–139

Soybeans and soy products, 68–69
 as source of plant protein, 68
 phytoestrogens in, 68–69

Spinach:
 nutritional benefits, 25–26

Starches:
 primary cause of weight gain, 15
 reducing intake, 121–122

restricted in Cayce diet, 11, 15

Steaming vegetables, *see also* Cooking
  methods
  to preserve nutrients, 40

Stress response, 111–118
  breathing, 100. *See also* Breathing
  how to improve, 123–124
  meditation, 111–112
  stress-free eating, 113–114

Stretching, 100–102. *See also* Exercise
  during exercise, 101–102

Supplements, nutritional, 124–127
  food-sourced, 124
  herbal tonics (Cayce formulations),
    126
  need for, 124–125

Sweeteners, 76–78
  beet sugar:
    recommended in Cayce
      readings, 77
  date sugar, 76–77
  honey, 77
  Sucanat, 76
  whole vs. refined, 76–78

T

Thermogenic foods:
  definition, 10

Thomas, Nancy, xiii, 84

Tomatoes:
  canned preferred, if not vine-
    ripened, 49. *See also* Canning
  nutritional value, 49

Turkey, 65. *See also* Poultry

V

Vegetable juices, fresh, *see also*
  Vegetables
  alkaline-forming, 13

fasts with, 106–107
Vegetables:
  above and below ground, 52–53
  canning to preserve, 48–49
  cruciferous, 32–34
    anticarcinogenic properties, 32
    how to prepare, 34
    nutritional benefits, 32–34
  drying to preserve, 50–51
  fermenting to preserve, 51
  freezing to preserve, 49–50
  green leafy:
    antioxidant properties, 23–24
    chlorophyll occurring in, 24
    how to prepare, 15. *See also* Cooking
      methods
  how to store, 46–47
  increasing intake, 120–121
  locally grown:
    benefits, 51–52
  nutritional benefits, 14–15
  organically grown, *see also*
    Organically grown foods
    benefits, 53–57
    higher nutrient content, 54–55
  recipes, 145–147
  sea vegetables, *see* Sea vegetables
  yellow and orange vegetables:
    antioxidant properties, 23–24
    nutrients occurring in, 24

W

Walking, 95–98. *See also* Exercise
  benefits, 95
  exercises during, recommended, 99
  increases fat-burning ability, 95–96
  lowers blood pressure, 97
  on treadmill, 97
  recommended for weight loss, 19

Water, 17–22
  and exercise:
    weight loss promoted by, 19
  benefits, 14, 17–22
  distilled, 21–22
  drinking water:
    types available, 19–21
    with added lemon juice, 21
  inadequate intake:

   health problems created by, 18
increased intake:
   how to implement, 120
   recommended for health
     conditions, 18–19
   weight loss promoted by, 18
   required for digestion and
     metabolism, 18

Watercress:
   nutritional benefits, 25
   prepared with gelatin, 25

Weight loss, affirmation for, 127

Weight-loss diets:
   Atkins, 6

   ineffectiveness of, 10
   low-carbohydrate:
     effective due to increased
      protein, 58
   number of people using, 6
   Ornish, 6
   South Beach, 7–9
   Zone, 6

Wine. *See* Red wine

Y

Yogurt, *see also* Lactic acid bacteria; Milk
   how to store, 63–64
   supports weight-loss efforts, 62

EDGAR CAYCE'S A.R.E.

What Is A.R.E.?

The Association for Research and Enlightenment, Inc., (A.R.E.®) was founded in 1931 to research and make available information on psychic development, dreams, holistic health, meditation, and life after death. As an open-membership research organization, the A.R.E. continues to study and publish such information, to initiate research, and to promote conferences, distance learning, and regional events. Edgar Cayce, the most documented psychic of our time, was the moving force in the establishment of A.R.E.

Who Was Edgar Cayce?

Edgar Cayce (1877–1945) was born on a farm near Hopkinsville, Ky. He was an average individual in most respects. Yet, throughout his life, he manifested one of the most remarkable psychic talents of all time. As a young man, he found that he was able to enter into a self-induced trance state, which enabled him to place his mind in contact with an unlimited source of information. While asleep, he could answer questions or give accurate discourses on any topic. These discourses, more than 14,000 in number, were transcribed as he spoke and are called "readings."

Given the name and location of an individual anywhere in the world, he could correctly describe a person's condition and outline a regimen of treatment. The consistent accuracy of his diagnoses and the effectiveness of the treatments he prescribed made him a medical phenomenon, and he came to be called the "father of holistic medicine."

Eventually, the scope of Cayce's readings expanded to include such subjects as world religions, philosophy, psychology, parapsychology, dreams, history, the missing years of Jesus, ancient civilizations, soul growth, psychic development, prophecy, and reincarnation.

A.R.E. Membership

People from all walks of life have discovered meaningful and life-transforming insights through membership in A.R.E. To learn more about Edgar Cayce's A.R.E. and how membership in the A.R.E. can enhance your life, visit our Web site at EdgarCayce.org, or call us toll-free at 800-333-4499.

Edgar Cayce's A.R.E.
215 67th Street
Virginia Beach, VA 23451–2061

EDGARCAYCE.ORG